HIV and AIDS
Your Questions Answered

OTHER TITLES IN THE SERIES
Your Questions Answered

Contraception - Your Questions Answered 2nd Edition
by John Guillebaud ISBN 0443 04070 2

Hormone Replacement Therapy - Your Questions Answered
by Malcolm Whitehead and Val Godfree ISBN 0443 04353 1

Anxiety and Depression - Your Questions Answered
by Cosmo Hallström and Nicola McClure ISBN 0443 04939 4

Arthritis and Rheumatism - Your Questions Answered
by Andrei Calin and John Cormack ISBN 0443 04988 2

HIV and AIDS
Your Questions Answered

By

Graham Barter
General Practitioner
Medical Director, Griffin Project
Continuing Care Unit, London, UK

Simon Barton
Consultant Genitourinary Physician,
St Stephen's Clinic, Chelsea and
Westminster Hospital, London, UK

Brian Gazzard
Consultant Physician,
St Stephen's Clinic, Chelsea and
Westminster Hospital, London, UK

Foreword by

Nick Partridge
The Terrence Higgins Trust,
London, UK

CHURCHILL LIVINGSTONE
EDINBURGH LONDON MADRID MELBOURNE NEW YORK AND TOKYO 1993

CHURCHILL LIVINGSTONE
Medical Division of Longman Group UK Limited

Distributed in the United States of America by
Churchill Livingstone Inc., 650 Avenue of the Americas, New York,
NY 10011, and by associated companies, branches and
representatives throughout the world.

First published 1993

ISBN 0-443-04752-9

British Library Cataloguing in Publication Data
A catalogue record for this book is available
from the British Library

Library of Congress Cataloging in Publication Data
is available

Typeset by Datix International Limited, Bungay, Suffolk
Printed in Great Britain at the University Press, Cambridge

Contents

Foreword

For many people, living with AIDS or HIV also means living with considerable uncertainty. The complexity of HIV infection means that you cannot be sure whether or when you may become ill or indeed with what. The long but unpredictable length of time between initial infection and first illness poses the first of many as yet unanswered questions about HIV. Why do some people become ill quickly and yet others stay well? More importantly, what can people living with HIV and their clinician do to maintain good health, and what are the first signs of impending illness?

With the continuing spread of HIV affecting a growing diversity of people, these questions and many others will be asked in surgeries and hospital consulting rooms with increasing frequency. Furthermore, there are over fifty opportunistic infections associated with AIDS, making it one of the most complex and difficult illnesses to live with or treat.

To make matters worse, since its arrival, AIDS has been surrounded by fear, prejudice and discrimination. Many of those first affected were already marginalized by medical perceptions of homosexuality, illegal drug use or their colour. One immediate result of this has been that many people with HIV have chosen not to involve their general practitioner in their primary care, through fear of yet another rejection or concern that their GP may simply not know what to do.

As a result, many people with HIV continue to travel considerable distances to increasingly overstretched centres of excellence for primary care and monitoring which can and should be provided locally. The reforms currently sweeping through (or possibly sweeping away) the National Health Service will hasten this process, as will the impact of the Tomlinson Report, should it be implemented, for currently over 70% of people with AIDS receive their treatment in central London.

These developments could create real risks for people with HIV seeking support and care in the future. If the knowledge, experience and understanding of AIDS is not developed as rapidly as legislative change is devolving services, then GPs and local hospitals will be left unprepared and people with HIV may suffer preventable illness as a result.

The St Stephen's Clinic of the Chelsea and Westminster Hospital, London, is one of the leading centres of excellence in Europe and has pioneered new models of care for people with HIV since the beginning of this epidemic. For many years now, the Clinic has run courses to encourage GPs and other health professionals to become involved in AIDS care. It is only through these initiatives that accessible, effective community care for people with HIV can become a reality.

This book, with its clear question and answer format, comes from experience often painfully gained over the past ten years. All too often AIDS continues to appear unnecessarily frightening though no longer because of its newness and apparent unpredictability, but because of its scope and scale. Furthermore, the intense media battle over AIDS, always contradictory and played out with the sound of personal axes being ground, has helped no one and confused many. Tragically, those hardest hit most recently have been HIV-positive health-care professionals who have had to cope not only with a life-threatening virus but also with the constant threat of vilification in the press.

It is this background which marks the importance of a book which covers the epidemiology, virology and immunology of HIV, as well as the counselling, treatment and multifaceted care needs of people living with AIDS. Sadly though, it is a measure of the challenges we all face that, even with considerable experience and extensive research, AIDS continues to pose complex questions and ethical dilemmas which have yet to be answered.

1993   N.P.

Preface

The aim of this book is to provide an accessible and comprehensible guide to the subject of human immunodeficiency virus (HIV) infection and acquired immunodeficiency syndrome (AIDS). Although this is a complex and fast moving field, every effort has been made to keep the information as up to date as possible and, where relevant, to point out the discrepancies in our knowledge and the direction for future research.

Many of the questions have emerged from our experiences in lecturing groups of doctors and other health professionals, especially at our regular St Stephen's, and Chelsea and Westminster Hospital AIDS courses. We thank the hundreds of General Practitioners who have attended these courses and contributed, by their interested and critical questioning, to the formulation of this book.

We thank our colleagues for their support in preparing this book. In particular, Dr Kate Pugh for contributing Chapter 10 on psychiatry and HIV infection, and Drs Surinder Singh and Simon Mansfield whose contribution to Chapter 17 on ethical dilemmas is duly acknowledged.

We would like to thank Philippa Blackhall for preparing the manuscript in meticulous style and Katia Chrysostomou for her support and cajoling to get us to complete this project.

Finally, we would like to acknowledge the enormous contribution of all our patients to this book. They provide the incentive and the inspiration to continue to strive for better understanding, therapy and support for everyone affected by HIV infection and AIDS.

London   G.B.
1993   S.B.
     B.G.

1. Epidemiology

1.1 Is it mainly homosexuals who become infected with HIV and develop AIDS?

Although AIDS was first recognized in the gay community in San Francisco in 1981, it rapidly became clear that this was a sexually transmitted disease which could affect any sexually active member of society. In addition, HIV could be transmitted by blood and therefore, before routine testing of blood for the virus became available, blood transfusion recipients and haemophiliacs were at increased risk of infection. Now the most rapidly growing group of patients with AIDS in the USA are those with heterosexually-acquired disease, and when one recognizes that this reflects acquisition of the virus 10 or more years ago, there is little doubt that heterosexually-transmitted AIDS is going to be the major problem in the USA in the next decade. Heterosexually-acquired AIDS is already very common throughout Europe, particularly in Spain and Italy.

Another major cause of transmission is the sharing of equipment by intravenous drug users. Sudden explosive increases in the incidence of HIV infection can occur in such communities. This was demonstrated in the early 1980s in Edinburgh and has since been witnessed in Bangkok. Partners of intravenous drug users often acquire HIV either sexually, or by sharing injecting equipment.

1.2 Will there be a large heterosexual outbreak of HIV infection in the UK?

The answer to this question is not known with certainty. There are definitely increasing numbers of patients in the UK who have acquired HIV heterosexually. The main risk for the heterosexual community is intravenous drug users, some of whom work in the sex industry to support their drug habit. Additionally, bisexual men may cause heterosexual spread of infection.

The size of any heterosexual epidemic is critically dependent on the frequency of partner change. Although rapid partner change is relatively common in the early years of sexual activity, this becomes less common after the age of 30, and so an epidemic is particularly likely in the younger age group.

1.3 What is the real scale of the epidemic — is it really true that everyone is threatened by HIV?

Some years ago, it was said that HIV infection was the major public health problem facing the world. This remains true today.

Globally, there are three patterns to the epidemic. Firstly, that seen in North America, Europe and Australia, where the disease was initially seen in the gay community and then spread via blood donation and intravenous drug use to heterosexuals and, to a lesser extent, children.

The second pattern of disease occurs in large parts of Oceania and Asia where the disease is, at present, relatively uncommon and has been introduced by travellers and through blood transfusion. Nevertheless, it is in this community that the next major explosive phase of the epidemic may well occur. For example, there has been a sudden marked rise in the incidence of HIV infection in the large population of female prostitutes in Bombay, from 0% in 1988 to over 40% in 1991. It is calculated that perhaps up to 1000 men per month are being infected in Bombay alone by this route.

Although the prevalence of HIV infection in countries following pattern two is currently low, the numbers who may develop AIDS there in the near future is high because of the enormous size of the population.

The third pattern of the epidemic is occurring in sub-Saharan Africa where transmission is primarily heterosexual, and vertical transmission is also common. A substantial proportion (10–60%) of the sexually active population of a number of urban communities are now infected with HIV. The rate of infection in the rural community is much lower. The premature deaths in urban society have a marked effect upon the financial structure of these developing nations, as those most affected are often the educated members of the community on whom the infrastructure of the society depends. The epidemic in this part of Africa is sufficiently large to influence demographic trends over the next 20 years, and no net population growth is expected in these communities.

The World Health Organization predicts that by the year 2000 there will be a cumulative total of 30 million people infected with HIV, 3 million of whom will have been infected within the last 3 years of the century. Of the total, 90% will be in developing countries. Ten million of the infections will be in children, and a further 10 million children, although not themselves infected, will be orphaned because of the premature death of both parents from AIDS.

1.4 What are the common methods of homosexual transmission?

A number of studies have shown that the risk is greatest with passive anal intercourse. This is quite frequently traumatic, and therefore HIV-infected semen gains direct access to the blood circulation of the recipient. Active penetrative sex is much less dangerous.

1.5 Is there any risk at all with oral sex?

The risk with oral sex is very low. There are several case reports of apparent HIV transmission via oral sex, but these are so infrequent that it is difficult to exclude other modes of transmission. Nevertheless, most safer sex advice continues to dissuade people from indulging in oral sex, or to use a dental dam or wear a flavoured condom.

1.6 Is there any particular sort of heterosexual activity which is more likely to cause transmission of HIV infection?

Most HIV transmission occurs during vaginal intercourse with an apparently 'healthy' looking partner. A number of studies have shown that certain factors increase the risk of transmission. One consistent factor is a history of venereal disease, because inflammation, ulceration or other genital lesions may facilitate transmission of the virus during sex.

As with homosexual sex, anal intercourse is another risk factor but only accounts for a small proportion of the total number of heterosexual HIV transmissions.

1.7 Do men or women acquire HIV more easily?

HIV, like all other venereal infections, is more easily acquired by a woman from a man than vice versa. Taking the contraceptive pill, which produces cervical ectropion exposing the fragile endocervix, may favour the acquisition of HIV during vaginal intercourse. Women with cervical infection, particularly chlamydia, may also be at increased risk, perhaps because of greater numbers of lymphocytes in cervical secretions.

In men, as with other venereal infections, being uncircumcized increases the risk of HIV acquisition. Genital ulcer disease also appears to be associated with a much increased transmission of HIV. Indeed, in one African study, over 50% of uncircumcized men who had a genital ulcer and visited a prostitute on one occasion became HIV infected (the prostitutes in this area had an 85% seroprevalence of HIV positivity).

1.8 What is the overall risk of becoming HIV infected after one episode of unprotected heterosexual intercourse?

It is difficult to estimate this risk accurately, but it is probably less than 1%. It may be much higher in Africa because of the high frequency of genital ulcer disease such as chancroid.

The risk of transmission is likely to be different at various stages of the disease. At the time of seroconversion, when rapid viral replication associated with the appearance of viral antigen in the circulation (p24) occurs, transmission of HIV appears particularly likely. Also, it may be more likely in patients just preceding AIDS development who again have more rapid viral replication. Thus in Africa, the majority of partners of AIDS patients are themselves HIV infected, while it is quite common for partners of HIV-positive well patients to be uninfected.

1.9 Can anything be done to reduce the risk of heterosexual acquisition of HIV?

Abstinence from sex provides complete protection against HIV by sexual transmission. If the previous sexual history of a partner is known to be with healthy uninfected people, HIV transmission is also less likely. Barrier methods of contraception probably reduce the risk of HIV transmission; the most effective of these appears to be the condom. Although condoms prevent the transmission of HIV during sexual intercourse, they may break. Condoms made of sheep's latex are more likely to be leaky, and may not prevent transmission. Female condoms such as Femidoms are now becoming available and are also likely to be protective. Caps which cover the whole cervical os may also offer some degree of protection. Spermicides are inhibitory to HIV, but do not offer sufficient protection to be used alone.

Although there are small studies demonstrating that people who use condoms regularly are at reduced risk of HIV infection, no large-scale studies conclusively demonstrating a reduced risk have been performed.

1.10 Is it absolutely certain that blood transfusion and the use of blood products are now not associated with transmission of HIV?

The method used when preparing factor concentrates and immunoglobulin now ensures that there is no risk from these products at all, as the virus will be inactivated during the process.

However, a tiny theoretical risk for blood transfusion remains. Early in the UK epidemic, perhaps 1 in 20 000 units of blood was infected. This was always much lower than in the USA, because UK policy does not allow payment for blood donations, and volunteer blood had a much lower chance of being HIV contaminated.

In this country, all blood is now tested for HIV-1 antibodies, and the blood transfusion service is constantly vigilant for a rise in the incidence of HIV-2, so that it could also be tested for very rapidly. Nevertheless, there is a theoretical risk of patients donating blood during the short period when virus is actively replicating but no antibody has yet been demonstrated. The risk that actual transmission of HIV by this mechanism will occur is very low, although it has been demonstrated in one case. Most patients in high-risk groups have voluntarily stopped donating blood, and patients who are viraemic, therefore particularly likely to be infectious, probably feel unwell and do not donate blood at this time.

1.11 Is it possible to reduce the risk of intravenous drug users acquiring HIV?

Intravenous drug users often come from underprivileged groups within society and have extremely poor access to healthcare facilities. This same group tends to be resistant to conventional advice. More success has been achieved by out-reach groups, which employ ex-users who contact current users to impart important public health messages and encourage individuals to attend for healthcare.

The most important healthcare message for people who continue to use drugs intravenously is that equipment should not be shared. In an emergency, the use of bleach and thorough cleaning of the needle and syringes probably does prevent the transfer of HIV. Needle exchange schemes are widely accepted now in the UK and much of Europe, but remain controversial in the USA because of unfounded fears of encouraging drug use. It is difficult to show conclusively that such exchanges do reduce transmission of HIV. The sharing of equipment seems to be reduced in those individuals using exchanges. They also seem to have better access to healthcare. Some innovative schemes of needle exchange in general practice have been tried with great success, and pharmacies also provide an important outlet for this activity. Drug users are in urgent need of advice about safe sexual activity to prevent the transfer of HIV to their partners, as well as clean needle exchange.

1.12 Are we certain that casual transmission of HIV cannot occur?

It is always very difficult in medicine to say 'never', and this case is no exception. All one can say is that casual transmission of HIV has never been documented, and the biological properties of the virus make this extremely unlikely. Studies of family members where there has been no sexual contact, and of schools where a high proportion of pupils are HIV-infected haemophiliacs, have shown no unexpected transmissions over quite long follow-up periods. The relative infrequency of infection amongst healthcare workers dealing with large numbers of HIV-positive patients is also reassuring.

1.13 How likely is it that an individual will develop HIV following injury with a needle contaminated with the virus?

A number of large prospective studies have looked at the risk of seroconversion following needlestick and blood-splash injury. The risk of seroconversion after needlestick injury is low at 0.37%. The risk of blood contamination of intact skin or mucus membrane causing seroconversion is much less than this. Indeed, there are only five documented cases where this has occurred, and in several of these, other potential mechanisms for transfer existed.

This low risk of seroconversion will vary depending upon the amount of blood transferred. Nearly all the seroconversions occur with microtransfusions of blood, rather than with transfer of the minute amount of blood (0.03 ml) present in the hollow bore of a needle. Seroconversions following a solid sharp injury (e.g. scalpel blade) appear very infrequent.

It is likely, but not proven, that patients at more infectious stages of the disease (at seroconversion and just prior to AIDS) might transmit the virus more readily.

1.14 How long after a needlestick injury is it safe to assume that the healthcare worker has not been infected?

This is a difficult question to answer. Nearly all documented cases of seroconversion following this sort of injury have occurred within the first 3 months. In the occasional case with a longer incubation period, there has usually been a potential alternative explanation for acquisition of infection. Although the possibility of seroconversion is low, it does represent great psychological trauma to those individuals who are exposed, and it is important to reduce this 'worrying' time as much as possible. It would therefore seem reasonable to tell patients that they are virtually safe if they have a negative test at 3 months, and completely safe if they have a negative test at 6 months.

There must be a very slight worry that a small amount of virus becomes latent following a needlestick injury, and does not excite a seroconversion reaction. Whilst this possibility cannot be totally excluded, two long-term follow-up studies using the most sensitive technology available (polymerase chain reaction), in people who have suffered a needlestick injury, show that in none was there evidence of HIV infection without a serological response.

1.15 Is there anything the healthcare worker can do following a needlestick injury to minimize the risk of infection?

Obviously it is sensible to make the wound bleed freely and to wash it thoroughly. The role of antiretroviral drugs, such as zidovudine (AZT), as prophylaxis is controversial.

There is no direct evidence that antiretroviral drugs will reduce the risk of seroconversion, and there are several instances where seroconversion has occurred, despite administration of the drug within a few hours. AZT is potentially toxic, teratogenic and oncogenic. Nevertheless, the risks are probably slight, and there are limited animal experimental data to suggest that AZT given concurrently with retroviruses can suppress viraemia. In discussion with many healthcare workers, it is found that some are keen to take any measures, however unlikely they are to succeed, to reduce the risk of infection, whilst others are more philosophical, accepting that the small risk of AZT without clear benefit is not worth taking. Although a controlled study of AZT prophylaxis in needlestick injuries was mounted in an attempt to settle this issue, the study was abandoned because few patients were enrolled.

Animal experiments suggest that if AZT is to be administered, it should be as early as possible and in large doses. No-one knows how long treatment should be continued in order to suppress viraemia, but probably 1 g of AZT should be given as soon as possible, and 1 g given daily for 2–6 weeks subsequently.

1.16 Is it possible that HIV-infected healthcare workers could infect their patients?

This has certainly occurred with an HIV-positive dentist in the USA who infected five of his patients. Although a number of other studies have shown no instances of seroconversion in patients operated upon by HIV-positive surgeons, such reassuring information may be misleading, as many of the procedures were minor or were performed at a time when the surgeon was probably not particularly infectious. Certainly, the analogy with hepatitis B-infected surgeons indicates that transmission to patients is possible, and that certain individuals may be more likely to cause transmission than others.

Recent studies have shown that needlestick injuries during surgery are common, and that quite a high proportion of these could also potentially infect the patient as, following puncture of the HIV-seropositive surgeon's skin, the needle re-enters the wound. Although the risk to an individual following such an injury is absolutely minuscule, because of the very large number of operations performed each year, it has been calculated that a number of individuals in America might be expected to be infected by this route.

1.17 What precautions should therefore be taken to prevent HIV-positive healthcare workers from infecting their patients?

As it is important to maintain the confidence of healthcare workers who otherwise may not come forward for advice, it does not seem sensible to institute routine testing. Equally, patients have the right to expect the best possible standards of care and to be protected from the risks of infection from their doctors and carers. Thus, anyone who knows or suspects that he is HIV positive is required to take appropriate advice from an expert. In general, such individuals should not undertake invasive procedures, and for cases of doubt or difficulty, a committee has been recently set up to provide advice. Clearly if such advice is to be acceptable, it must be recognized that HIV infection may occur as a result of an occupational exposure and therefore be compensated for adequately.

2. Virology

2.1 What sort of virus is HIV?

HIV is a retrovirus. All viruses in this group are characterized by the presence of a unique enzyme, reverse transcriptase, which converts viral RNA into a DNA template called a provirus, which is then inserted in the genome of the host cell. Retroviruses include transforming viruses capable of causing tumours in animals (e.g. murine leukaemia virus), and lentiviruses which can produce an immunodeficiency state in animals similar to AIDS (e.g. simian immunodeficiency virus, SIV).

2.2 Can we be certain that HIV causes AIDS?

There is no doubt that HIV is the agent primarily responsible for AIDS. The evidence for this is overwhelming. Perhaps the single best evidence comes from transmission of AIDS to patients with no other obvious risk of infection other than a blood transfusion. HIV can be cultured from such patients and also from the blood of the original donor. As well as this epidemiological evidence, HIV as a cause of AIDS makes biological sense; similar viruses cause similar diseases in animals. HIV is known to infect and destroy CD4 lymphocytes (see Ch. 3) and a reduction in the CD4 lymphocyte count is a major feature of AIDS. Doubts about HIV as the only cause of AIDS have been expressed and given some credence, primarily because the rate of CD4 lymphocyte loss is difficult to explain on the basis of the number of cells infected at any one time. However, it is possible that uninfected cells are also destroyed because soluble virological products adhere to their surface, or because the body produces autoantibodies which destroy even uninfected CD4 lymphocytes. HIV being the major cause of AIDS does not preclude other infections, particularly viruses like human herpes virus 6 or Epstein–Barr virus from acting as cofactors. Such a cofactor may stimulate the regulatory genes of HIV and encourage it to replicate more rapidly.

2.3 Does the life cycle of HIV indicate any ways in which drug therapy may be used to inhibit the virus?

Areas on the virus envelope recognize the CD4 receptor on CD4 lymphocytes and other cells and allow the virus to come into intimate contact with the cell surface. The subsequent cell fusion events are complex and are now being elucidated. Although dextran sulphate inhibits this process, it is not absorbed when given orally. The addition of soluble CD4 into the circulation will confuse the virus and cause it to combine with the soluble product and prevent it from infecting cells. If soluble CD4 is present in the circulation, coupled to antibodies, then the resulting CD4–viral antibody complex may be destroyed by immune cells containing a special receptor responsive to antibody complexed to antigen called the Fc receptor. Despite the considerable ingenuity of this idea, human investigations using these products have been disappointing. This is partly because initial laboratory experiments gave misleading results. Laboratory forms of HIV have been selected because of their ease of growth in tissue cultures containing cells with CD4 receptors, while viruses actually cultured from patients have much less affinity to the CD4 receptor. Thus the ability of soluble CD4 to inhibit virus replication in vitro is not reproduced in vivo.

Reverse transcriptase is a unique enzyme which enables the manufacture of DNA from viral RNA. Inhibiting this enzyme would be expected to prevent viral replication while being relatively non-toxic to humans. Of the drugs presently available to treat HIV most belong to this class of compound (see Ch. 14).

The proviral DNA made by reverse transcriptase is formed into a circle prior to incorporation in the host genome. Theoretically, both processes could be interfered with, but no drug is nearing clinical production. Following incorporation in the host genome, unknown factors cause the production of viral regulatory gene products, most importantly Tat protein. This protein interacts with sequences at the edge of the proviral DNA sequence, called the long terminal repeats, and this interaction causes enhanced production of the viral structural proteins. This Tat protein has now been synthesized, and at least one drug potentially capable of inhibiting its action is in development. One of the factors which may prevent the virus from reproducing itself continuously is another viral gene product called Nef. Although the function of this protein remains controversial, many accept that it reduces viral replication. This may have a survival advantage for the virus by slowing down the speed of replication, allowing the host to live longer and making it more likely that the virus can disseminate to alternative hosts. Again it is possible that this Nef protein could be reproduced in a laboratory and used in HIV-positive patients to keep the virus suppressed.

An important viral enzyme, protease, cleaves the initial viral precursor protein products, producing the active compounds. This enzyme is different from mammalian proteases, it has been crystallized, and inhibitors have been produced. These inhibitors are at present in Phase 1 human trials.

2.4 Do any other viruses cause AIDS in human beings?

Yes. Another virus called HIV-2 was discovered in western Africa and more recently in parts of Latin America. HIV-2 is closely related to HIV-1, although HIV-2 has two extra regulatory genes compared with HIV-1, and there is a 20–30% dissimilarity in the amino acid sequences of the coat of the two viruses. HIV-2 is also closely related to SIV (which causes an AIDS-like illness in some species of monkeys). It is thought that HIV-2 and SIV originated from a single primate virus about a century ago. No primate virus with such a close similarity to HIV-1 has been described. It is therefore possible that HIV-1 has been present as an occasional infection in the human race for much longer than HIV-2. The latter is transmitted in the same way as HIV-1 and causes the same range of diseases, although it is possible that patients may develop AIDS rather more slowly.

Recently, reports of several individuals suffering from AIDS, with low CD4 lymphocyte counts, but who are seronegative for both HIV-1 and HIV-2 have caused concern. However, it is unlikely that this phenomenon represents evidence for a novel immunosuppressive virus.

2.5 What virological factors make it difficult to produce a vaccine against HIV?

HIV is covered with a sugar coat which may not be immunogenic. Only two small parts of the virus are exposed through this coat, the V3 loop and the CD4 receptor site. The CD4 receptor site may be very similar to human antigens which would be treated as 'self', thus inducing no immune response. The V3 loop is so named because it comes from a hyper-variable region of the genome. Within a few months of infection, multiple mutations have often occurred in this loop, and although initial antibodies produced by the patient to the loop neutralize the virus, several months after infection they do not. Antigenic variation of the envelope is thus one of the main reasons that vaccine development is likely to be slow. Wild type viruses isolated from individuals in different parts of the world vary in amino acid structure by up to 30%. Recent data from Bangkok indicate that individuals may have widely different antigenic determinants on the surface of their particular virus, although all patients come from a confined locality.

The ability of the virus to remain latent means that little or no viral products are produced for long periods. Latently-infected cells may have no surface signal to indicate the presence of HIV. Such cells cannot be destroyed by the immune system as they are not recognized to be harbouring the virus.

2.6 Are there factors of viral virulence which influence the rapidity of AIDS development?

This is a controversial subject, but it is clear that the virus isolated early in the disease replicates more slowly and is less cytopathic than the virus which is isolated from patients late in disease. This latter stage virus also infects CD4 cells more easily than macrophages, and is more likely to produce syncytia of these lymphocytes thereby increasing the rate of CD4 lymphocyte destruction. If this rapidly replicating form of virus infects another person, the virus tends to revert to a more slowly replicating form, presumably because of host control mechanisms. Nevertheless, it is believed that one of the few factors besides age which influences the speed of development of AIDS, is being infected by a patient with more advanced disease with one of these viruses which may be more virulent. It has also been suggested that this virulent form or syncytial inducing strain is less responsive to antiviral therapy.

2.7 Does viral resistance to drugs develop during treatment, and if so, what is its importance?

When virus is isolated from HIV-infected patients who have been treated for a year or more with AZT, it is less sensitive to the drug in tissue culture experiments (so-called resistance). Virus isolated from the individuals prior to treatment will always be sensitive to AZT. Viral resistance to AZT requires four or five separate mutations within the reverse transcriptase gene. This part of the viral genome is relatively conserved, i.e. most mutations in this area of the gene are lethal to the virus and so mutations of this sort are much slower to emerge. Interestingly, viruses with resistance to AZT remain sensitive to other dideoxynucleosides, in particular dideoxyinosine (ddI) and dideoxycytosine (ddC). There is, however, cross resistance between AZT resistance and the closely related drug, AZDU. More recently, a mutation which produces resistance to ddI has been described. This mutation produces cross resistance to ddC. However, it is of considerable potential importance that viruses known to be resistant to AZT cultured from patients treated with ddI, become sensitive to AZT again as ddI resistance emerges. Such AZT-sensitive viruses contain the mutations for resistance to both AZT and ddI, i.e. the mutation producing resistance to ddI makes the AZT-resistant virus sensitive again.

Resistance has also been described to the new allosteric inhibitors of reverse transcriptase (the Tibol compounds). Such resistant forms only require two mutations and seem to develop rapidly.

There is as yet no correlation between clinical progression of disease and viral resistance. There is a clinical impression, not substantiated by any studies, that AZT becomes less effective after 1–2 years' treatment, and it is certainly during this period that viral resistance becomes commonplace. It could be, however, that AZT-resistant strains are less virulent. This is certainly true of the herpes viruses that become resistant to acyclovir. Nonetheless, most clinicians would believe that it is highly likely that viral resistance is associated with loss of clinical effectiveness of AZT, and is one of the main reasons why the use of combination drugs which may prevent the development of such resistance is becoming a popular idea.

3. Immunology

3.1 What antibody response does the patient make to HIV infection?

As with any other viral infection, after about 2–3 weeks an antibody response occurs in the patient, which is initially of IgM antibody class and subsequently of IgG. Production of these antibodies is stimulated by the various constituents of the virus, the two most important being the core and the surface. Surface antibody (anti-gp120), which is detected by the enzyme-linked immunosorbent assay (ELISA) commonly employed to indicate HIV infection, is maintained until the patient's death. However, the titre of core antibody (p24 antibody) tends to wane as the infection progresses. Indeed, this may be one of the factors which predicts the development of AIDS.

3.2 Is there a cellular immune response to HIV infection?

In addition to humoral immunity, a cellular immune response also arises from HIV infection. Lymphocytes are now distinguished using monoclonal antibodies which recognize different surface receptors. The two broad categories are B lymphocytes, which develop into antibody-producing cells, and T lymphocytes, which provide cell-mediated immunity. One type of T lymphocyte is the CD4 lymphocyte, or so-called helper cell, which enhances the immune response through the production of many locally acting hormones or cytokines. Another T lymphocyte, the CD8 lymphocyte, has two distinct functions; some act as specific killer cells destroying cells infected with viruses, whilst others suppress the immune response of the patient which is important once an infection has been successfully overcome.

As HIV gains entry to cells via the CD4 receptor, it is not surprising that progressive HIV infection is accompanied by a loss of these cells. Initially, however, there is a strong CD8 lymphocyte, or killer cell, response which reduces the replication rate of the virus.

3.3 Why, if there is an initial good immune response to HIV infection, do patients go on to develop AIDS?

This is one of the central conundrums of HIV infection. Initially, patients produce a neutralizing antibody directed mainly against a variable portion of the envelope called the V3 loop. Owing to rapid antigenic mutation (see Ch. 2) the virus begins to evade this neutralizing antibody. However, different variants of HIV are probably controlled for much longer by the cellular immune system.

One of the theories for AIDS development from HIV infection is termed 'antigenic diversity'; the theory being that progressive mutations are controlled by the immune system until there are so many that the immune system fails.

The onset of AIDS is obviously preceded by a marked reduction in the CD4 lymphocyte count. It remains controversial whether this count drops gently in the majority of patients throughout the course of their illness, or is stable and falls suddenly prior to the onset of AIDS. It is possible that both mechanisms occur in different patients.

As well as a falling CD4 lymphocyte count, there also appear to be specific defects in CD4 lymphocyte function which predict the development of AIDS, e.g. the ability to respond by proliferation to certain monoclonal antibodies (anti-CD3). The functional abnormalities of CD4 lymphocytes are measured clinically by a failure of delayed hypersensitivity skin reactions, e.g. the tuberculin test.

As well as failure of CD4 lymphocyte functions, specific CD8 lymphocyte function is also inhibited. Thus, killing of cytomegalovirus (CMV)-infected cells is deficient in HIV-infected individuals, even though the CD8 lymphocytes are present in normal numbers. Similarly, although the number of monocytes/macrophages is normal in HIV-seropositive patients, they fail to control certain infections. A laboratory test for this cell type is analysis of the ability to kill *Toxoplasma gondii*-infected cells. The failure of CD8 lymphocytes and cells of the monocyte lineage can be partially corrected by the addition of cytokines, e.g. interleukin-2, which are normally produced by the CD4 lymphocytes and thus may be a secondary phenomenon caused by HIV infection of CD4 lymphocytes. However, macrophages which also have CD4 surface receptors are themselves infected with HIV which may interfere with their function. Macrophage infection may also be a long-term reservoir for HIV release, as the virus can replicate in these cells without causing lysis. Macrophage infection also stimulates the production of a variety of cytokines which have important physiological functions, like dilatation of blood vessels and encouragement of fibrogenesis. This may explain some of the unusual effects of HIV infection, such as the frequent occurrence of Kaposi's sarcoma — a vascular tumour.

3.4 I don't understand why, if only small numbers of T lymphocytes are infected with HIV, the numbers fall so quickly during HIV infection. Could you explain?

This puzzle has led some observers to believe that HIV is not the cause of AIDS. However, sophisticated mathematical modelling indicates that the number of CD4 lymphocytes known to be infected with HIV (between 1:100 and 1:1000 in advanced disease) is enough to account for the CD4 lymphocyte decline over a period of years. As well as direct cytotoxicity, additional mechanisms for the fall in CD4 lymphocyte count may also be important. Many soluble products of virus are liberated from infected cells into the circulation. Products like gp120, the envelope protein, may attach to other CD4 lymphocytes. These cells may then in turn be attacked by the immune system because they have on their surface a signal (gp120) which is recognized as foreign. gp120 attached to the surface of cells may also combine with the CD4 receptor on uninfected cells, producing large syncytia. Virus producing syncytia in vitro occurs in late-stage disease and this is one of the phenotypic features of rapidly replicating virus strains. Such syncytia, although rarely seen in man, commonly occur in various animals infected with retroviruses.

3.5 Why do conditions in the mouth and the skin so often herald the onset of AIDS?

There is no clear answer to this important question. There are more immunologically competent cells in the gut and skin than anywhere else in the body. Together they form the mucocutaneous immune system which is very often the first line of defence against infection. It is interesting how many of the opportunistic infections of AIDS infect these tissues, e.g. *Pneumocystis carinii* pneumonia, cryptosporidiosis and oesophageal candidiasis. Normally, antigens gain access to the circulation through specific cells (m cells) in the gut situated in Peyer's patches. This stimulates the production of T and B lymphocytes which circulate around the body, but preferentially re-congregate in the mucocutaneous immune system, because a special receptor causes them to attach to venules in the skin and mucus membranes.

Clinical evidence of a failure of the mucocutaneous immune system is nearly always a premonitory feature of AIDS. Thus more than half the patients who have oral candidiasis will have developed AIDS within 1 year. The risk of developing AIDS is also heightened in patients who have multidermatomal herpes zoster. Many other skin infections are also more common during this 'transitory' phase of HIV infection.

3.6 What immune functions should be monitored during HIV infection and how frequently?

Probably the most important test and certainly the one that the patient will be most aware of, is a count of the number of CD4 lymphocytes. It should be recognized that measurement of this is subject to quite wide laboratory error, and it is important that samples be analysed in a laboratory with good standards of quality control. It is also important that no therapeutic action should be taken on the basis of one sample, but only after two samples have produced congruent results. Much of the variability in CD4 lymphocyte numbers is due to changes in the total lymphocyte count. Therefore, there is now a move to rely more on CD4 lymphocyte percentages — but these are less familiar to most clinicians.

There is a very wide range of normal CD4 lymphocyte counts and it probably varies slightly with the time of the day and with age. A lower normal limit of between 350 and 500 cells/mm³ is set by most laboratories but this is an arbitrary range, and most patients have CD4 lymphocyte counts which are considerably above this. In the early stages of the disease when the CD4 lymphocyte count is high, it is probably only important to measure the count once or twice a year. In later stages of the disease, patients may wish to begin therapy when the CD4 lymphocyte count falls below certain predetermined limits (see Ch. 14), and therefore more frequent counts, perhaps every 3 months, are necessary. CD4 lymphocyte counts retain a prognostic value even after a diagnosis of AIDS; however, in late disease when the CD4 lymphocyte count is low (below 50 cells/mm³), minor changes are probably not clinically important and therefore the count needs to be performed less frequently.

Whilst a good functional measure of the CD4 lymphocyte count is to look at skin delayed hypersensitivity reactions, repetition of these tests may induce reappearance of responses and so they are not widely performed. Also, some patients, even with advanced AIDS, retain a positive tuberculin reaction.

Other tests of the immune system include monitoring levels of β_2 microglobulin or neopterin in the circulation or urine, which signal the degree of activation of lymphocytes. Such tests also predict the development of AIDS with accuracy and are used extensively by some units.

3.7 Do other infections or vaccinations encourage more rapid AIDS development by antigenic stimulation?

As HIV is not actively replicating in the majority of infected CD4 lymphocytes, worries have been expressed that if these CD4 lymphocytes become activated, the rate of replication of the virus will be quicker, and thus AIDS develop more quickly.

Some antigens, such as bacterial toxins, are so-called super antigens because they stimulate CD4 lymphocytes directly without being processed by antigen-presenting cells. Professor Montagner believes that this is one way in which CD4 lymphocytes may diminish, as such activated cells are programmed to die by a mechanism known as apoptosis (see Qu. 3.8).

It is also possible that other virus infections which might themselves infect T lymphocytes can produce activation of the cells and thus cause replication of HIV. Candidates for this form of interactive infection include human herpes virus 6. Another cofactor which, it has been suggested, accelerates the rate at which AIDS develops is infection with mycoplasma. These are common laboratory contaminants and their role as cofactors in HIV-infected patients is still controversial.

Thus, it is possible that a variety of coinfections might accelerate the development of AIDS, but it appears very difficult to know how to avoid such infections. Fortunately, advice about safe sexual practices for an HIV-positive individual also protects the individual from acquiring a variety of venereal infections, which are amongst the most likely cofactors to have a role in accelerating the development of AIDS.

There is no clear evidence that treatment of any of these putative cofactors might reduce the rapidity of AIDS onset. Part of the controversy surrounding coinfection is that many eminent scientists do not wish a research effort against HIV to be misdirected towards a search for treatable cofactors, which at best can only slow down the rate at which AIDS will develop.

Antigenic stimulation by vaccine could also activate T lymphocytes and encourage more rapid viral replication. However, reviews of HIV-seropositive children who have been inadvertently vaccinated with live and dead vaccines show no evidence of increased progression.

3.8 Could you say a little more about apoptosis?

Programmed cell death is a normal phenomenon occurring in immature thymocytes, in which cells die as nuclease enzymes split the DNA into oligonucleotides. This phenomenon can be increased by calcium ionophores, by antigen processed by antigen presenting cells, or by certain antigens (super antigens) without the help of these cells. Apoptosis is increased in HIV-positive patients. In some cases up to 40% of lymphocytes may undergo programmed cell death when stimulated by super antigen or mitogen. The reason for this increased responsiveness is unknown, as is the relevance of this phenomenon in the progression to AIDS, but it may be that repeated stimulation with different antigens leads to eradication of clones of lymphocytes capable of responding to these antigens with consequent progressive immune deficit.

3.9 How likely are we to see a vaccine against HIV appearing in the next few years?

Many properties of HIV make the production of a vaccine difficult. Marked antigenic variation in parts of the viral envelope allow the virus to evade the effects of neutralizing antibody. There are conserved areas within the envelope, but unfortunately it may be more difficult to raise a vaccine against these, and induction of an antibody which can prevent infection may also be less likely. Although such neutralizing antibody is produced by the host during the course of HIV infection, it does not prevent progressive infection.

The second problem is that HIV infects the very cells which will be responsible for the production of the vaccine response, i.e. the antigen-presenting cells (macrophages) and the CD4 lymphocytes.

The third problem is that HIV is an intracellular infection which may be transmitted from cell to cell without exposure to the plasma containing neutralizing antibody. This cell to cell transmission may be particularly important in the initial phase of infection.

The fourth major difficulty to be overcome is the latency of HIV infection. HIV becomes irreversibly incorporated in the genome of various cells, and such cells may have no surface evidence of their infection. These cells will therefore never be eradicated by the immune system because they will not be recognized as 'foreign'.

Yet a further difficulty surrounding the development of a successful vaccine is that some potential vaccines have produced enhancing antibody. This is a form of antibody which actually increases the ability of HIV to infect new cells, at least in tissue culture. Such antibody could coat HIV-infected cells without destroying them, and by doing so expose the Fc receptor. Thus cells which recognize the Fc receptor can come into intimate contact with an HIV-infected cell, and become infected in turn. The possibility of enhancing functions, which have so far been demonstrated with antibodies to gp41 (one of the envelope proteins), is particularly important if vaccines are to be used in HIV-infected individuals to stimulate an increased immune response in the hope of eradicating infection.

Various vaccine approaches have been tried using small segments of the virus envelope. There has been little success. A whole envelope vaccine, either a gp120 or gp160 has been used with more success. A vaccine using this approach has been successfully developed against simian immunodeficiency virus (SIV). Recent reports have raised doubts about the validity of some of these experiments, as injection of the cell lines used to grow the viruses also induced a protective response.

A gp160 vaccine has been shown to be safe in man and to produce antibodies. Testing that these vaccines have a protective function in man is a difficult undertaking and virtually impossible in the western world because of the very low rate of seroconversion. To test vaccines may be possible in the third world, but the ethics of such an undertaking are difficult, as such a programme could primarily benefit the western world, being too expensive to use in the third world. An obvious compromise would be that if a successful vaccine were developed it should be delivered free to such countries.

As live vaccines might incorporate undesirable parts of the HIV virus, less research has been done on this sort of vaccine, but some human studies have been done with vaccinia virus incorporating part of the HIV envelope.

The balance of evidence remains that a vaccine will be difficult to achieve and that it is unlikely that rapid progress will be made in the next 2 or 3 years, but in the 5–10 year period, the chances that an effective agent will be developed should improve.

3.10 Is it possible that immunostimulation might be an approach to the treatment of HIV infection?

One of the disappointing aspects of the use of antiretroviral agents is that although they reduce the rate of viral replication, there is only a small improvement in immune function, measured by sophisticated tests of CD4 lymphocyte activity or in total numbers of CD4 lymphocytes present in the circulation.

Several drugs are known to increase the numbers of circulating CD4 lymphocytes and sometimes to improve their function. These include levamisole, immunothiol and thymosin (a hormone derived from the thymus). Only immunothiol has been subjected to a controlled clinical trial, and patients taking this drug developed AIDS more rapidly than those taking placebo. This illustrates one of the worries of the use of immunostimulation as this may lead to more rapid viral replication unless an effective antiretroviral agent is used in addition to the im-munostimulant. Combinations of antiretrovirals and immunostimulants have not yet been used on a wide scale.

An alternative approach to immunostimulation is vaccination, as mentioned above. A vaccination programme for HIV-seropositive individuals with envelope vaccines (gp160) is in progress in the USA, and in some cases improvement of the immune system occurred. Additionally Salk, the discoverer of the polio vaccine, has used a formalin-killed vaccine where the coat of HIV has been removed, exposing core antigen. This vaccine has been used with some apparent improvement in immune function in infected patients. Support for vaccines which potentially improve prospects for HIV-positive individuals also comes from animal data. Cats with early infection with feline T-cell leukaemia virus (FTLV; a retrovirus with some similarities to HIV) were inoculated with a vaccine and were able to ablate the reservoir of FTLV infection, presumably by cytotoxic cells generated by the vaccine.

3.11 What is the autoimmune theory regarding the causation of AIDS?

It was noted early in the HIV epidemic that there was a similarity between some of the pathological features, particularly in the skin and gut and 'graft versus host disease'. This is a disease in which lymphocytes present in a tissue graft, like a kidney, attacked the host and caused immune damage. Part of the HIV envelope looks like major histocompatibility (MHC) class II antigen. It has therefore been suggested that this molecular mimicry may produce an immune response which, as well as being directed against the virus coat, produces an autoimmune attack on host cells expressing MHC class II antigens. Such homology might also explain why cell lines injected into macaque monkeys themselves produce protection from subsequent challenge by SIV, the hypothesis being that these cell lines produced an MHC class antibody response which prevented the subsequent SIV infection. The full theory is extremely complex, involving an understanding of the normal controlling mechanisms of the immune system via the anti-idiotype network. However, one of the advantages of this particular theory is that it does propose hypotheses which are relatively straightforward to test.

4. Prevention of HIV and infection control

4.1 What is the risk of an individual developing HIV infection following a needlestick injury from an HIV-seropositive patient?

Serial studies of healthcare workers who have received a needlestick injury involving a significant inoculation of known HIV-seropositive blood have shown the risk to be 0.37%. This figure is based on a 5-year follow-up of over 1000 healthcare workers. It would seem likely that the risk of HIV seroconversion, following exposure to HIV-seropositive blood via non-penetrating cutaneous or mucosal surface contamination, is likely to be considerably lower than this figure.

It has been suggested that several factors may increase the risk of HIV transmission during a needlestick injury. Firstly, the risk would increase with the volume of the inoculum and the quantity of virus inoculated into the recipient. This latter factor may be influenced by the stage of disease in the patient from which the blood originated (i.e. the risk may be higher if the patient had an active seroconversion illness, had developed AIDS, or had an associated high titre antigenemia). Secondly, deep penetration of blood will render it less accessible to simple washing and skin disinfection procedures, thus is likely to carry with it an increased transmission rate. Finally, it is possible, although unproven, that certain immunological and/or genetic factors in the recipient may determine the likelihood of infection.

4.2 Is AZT of any benefit following a needlestick injury?

This is a fine example of a clinical problem in which healthcare workers have not 'practised what they preach' — failing to participate in a double-blind randomized clinical control trial. Instead, individual institutions have developed their own policies for offering people, who arc the recipients of needlestick injuries from HIV-seropositive blood, AZT therapy in an attempt to reduce that individual's chances of infection. The data on which this is based come from experimental animals using viruses other than HIV-1. There are now several reports of people who received AZT within a few hours of undergoing a needlestick injury who have seroconverted and become HIV antibody positive. Furthermore, the possible short- and long-term side-effects experienced by healthcare workers who receive one or more courses of AZT following needlestick injuries are unclear.

Despite these uncertainties, many healthcare workers have opted to receive AZT and, in the absence of hard data on the efficacy of this treatment, many will continue to do so. It is vital that information from their experiences be collated and used in an attempt to define further protocols. Even more important is that all units involved in taking blood samples or engaging in surgical procedures on patients should have a clear policy on practise following a needlestick injury. This should involve immediate wound hygiene and irrigation, as well as immediate counselling on the options for the person who has undergone the accident. This should be provided by an experienced physician who has the ability to prescribe AZT and other types of prophylaxis if appropriate.

4.3 How should a health worker who has received a needlestick injury be managed?

The key to proper management of needlestick injuries is for each unit to have a properly thought-out, written and well-publicized policy prior to the needlestick injury occurring. Individual workers in healthcare and laboratory situations should have immediate access to named personnel who are able to deal with these problems. It is vital that provision is made within domestic, portering, and other support and hotel services staff for such incidents.

If you are the person to whom the exposed healthcare worker presents, it is vital to take a full history in order to categorize the exposure route into one of the following:

1. Direct transcutaneous exposure.
2. Mucus membrane inoculation.
3. Open skin wound contamination.
4. Contamination of intact skin.

In needlestick and other percutaneous incidents, it is important to describe the size and type of needle or other instrument involved, estimate the approximate depth of penetration, estimate the volume of blood injected, describe the site wound appearance, estimate the amount of bleeding produced, and state the time at which the exposure occurred. These details enable the degree of risk induced by the exposure event to be approximately calculated.

The exposed healthcare worker should be encouraged to undergo HIV antibody testing, or at the very least to have a serum sample banked as soon as possible after exposure has occurred. It should be explained to them that without a negative baseline HIV antibody test, proving that infection was temporarily related to the exposure event will be impossible, and this may have implications for the worker's ability to claim compensation. If an HIV antibody test is to be performed, it is vital that pre-test counselling includes a discussion of other possible risk factors as well as the issues which are routinely covered in pre-test counselling (see Ch. 5). Subsequent HIV antibody testing will usually be advised 2, 6 and 12 months after exposure. This sequential testing is useful in allaying fears of patients about delayed seroconversion as well as documenting continued seronegativity, and will only rarely result in diagnosing HIV infection. It is important that the subject of HIV does not lead to forgetting to examine the risk of the injured party from contracting other infections, e.g. hepatitis B, syphilis, etc. The prevention of both bacterial and viral infections by this route is vital.

As the majority of reported occupational episodes of HIV infection have been accompanied by symptoms of an acute seroconversion illness, exposed healthcare workers should be advised to report with any symptoms and signs of fever, lymphadenopathy, rash, headache, fatigue, etc. The use of HIV p24 antigen tests, viral cultures or polymerase chain reactions (PCR) in individual cases should be discussed between the laboratory and the individual physician before offering such tests to the patient.

It will be recommended that following a probable exposure risk to HIV-infected body fluids, healthcare workers should engage in safer sexual practises with their sexual partners to reduce the potential for transmission until a negative HIV antibody test at 6 months has ruled out infection. Unfortunately, this advice frequently produces confusion and anxiety in the exposed person and their sexual partners, and the role of trained counsellors to support the individuals and their families and lovers during this time is vital.

The role of AZT prophylaxis will only become an issue if people present early with needlestick injuries. Theoretically, the use of AZT or other nucleoside analogues administered soon after exposure might prevent HIV infection by obstructing HIV replication in the initial target cells. Animal studies suggest that protection is most apparent when treatment is started within 24 hours of exposure. The optimal dosage and duration of chemoprophylaxis has not been established, but most protocols employ doses of 250 mg 4 times a day for 2–6 weeks. The aim is to start chemoprophylaxis, if a significant risk has occurred and the exposed healthcare worker understands the absence of hard data, within as short a time as possible. This will not be achieved without good pathways of reporting needlestick injuries, pre-existent knowledge about action to be taken in the event of exposure to HIV-infected blood, and the availability of trained personnel at all times to deal with exposed healthcare workers.

4.4 What if the needlestick injury has occurred from a patient who is HIV untested but is thought to be at high risk of being HIV positive?

These patients will fall into two main groups. Firstly, the patient with symptoms and signs of HIV infection but who has not yet agreed to or been offered HIV antibody testing. Clearly, the advice of a physician experienced in managing patients with HIV infection should be sought for their opinion about the clinical likelihood of HIV infection in the individual case. If the patient is suffering from an AIDS-indicator illness, in the absence of any other obvious causes of immunosuppression, then for the management of the person who has been injured, their blood or body fluid should be treated as being HIV seropositive.

Secondly, the case of the person with no symptoms or signs of HIV infection or associated diseases, but who is known to have engaged in behaviour which would make them more likely to be at risk of acquiring HIV infection, e.g. a homosexual man, an injecting drug user or a haemophiliac who has received Factor VIII prior to 1985. The management of this group should be to inform them of the incident which has occurred, openly and totally non-judgementally. It is important to emphasize that it is not compulsory for them to have an HIV test, but to demonstrate, through simple discussion, the benefits this would have for the management of the person who has been exposed.

In the majority of cases the patient will usually accept the benefits for the healthcare worker and agree to be tested. It is important that pre-test counselling is offered to them in the standard way, so that the benefits to themselves of having an HIV antibody test can also be weighed up against any possible adverse effects. The patient's decision to have an HIV test will not directly impact on the initial management of the exposed healthcare worker. It is unlikely that the HIV test result would be available within the initial time in which they need to decide on the use of AZT chemoprophylaxis. However, the result will impact on the continuation of AZT therapy if started, and on the continued safer sexual practises, and levels of anxiety and psychological disturbances seen in the exposed healthcare worker.

4.5 Should an HIV-infected doctor continue to practise medicine?

In the UK the General Medical Council have written to every doctor reminding them of their responsibility — to ensure they do not place their patients at risk of infection. However, no enforceable ruling has been made on the level at which an HIV-infected doctor should or should not practise medicine or surgery. The logical way to approach this problem is threefold.

Firstly, the identification of HIV-antibody-positive doctors. There is no rule that doctors should be mandatorily tested. Some doctors, especially those who have had needlestick injuries, or who have perceived themselves to be at risk because of their professional or private lives, have undergone HIV antibody testing. As the results of these tests remain confidential, and as the majority of doctors have not been tested, it is clear that no assessment of the current prevalence of HIV infection amongst doctors in the UK, or indeed anywhere else in the world, exists at present.

Secondly, there is confusion about the level of risk which the infected doctor poses to a patient. Clearly, problems will arise if doctors perform procedures during which they are at risk of injuring themselves and causing spillage of blood into a body cavity, e.g. during surgery, or via a cannula during a percutaneous procedure. From what is known about the risk of the reverse situation, that is a doctor being infected from a patient, it is likely that the risk of a doctor injuring a patient in this way would be considerably less than 0.4%. However, the recent case of a Florida dentist with AIDS who appears to have infected five of his patients during routine dental practise is puzzling. Explanations of this cluster of surgeon-to-patient infections have not been readily forthcoming. Partly in view of this, it is strongly suggested that HIV-seropositive doctors or dentists who perform operative procedures should change their practise away from this work. Essentially, any procedure in which there is a possibility that doctors could injure themselves, in a situation which would cause blood to be passed inside their patient, should be avoided.

Thirdly, the question arises 'who is responsible once the decision to allow an HIV-infected doctor to continue practising is made?' If he/she consults a fellow professional or representative body and seeks advice, then if a patient were subsequently to be infected even though he/she followed their recommendations, there may be a risk of litigation. Such worries are currently being tested in courts in the USA, but as yet it is unclear what the British position on this matter would be. Unfortunately, what is certain is that an increasing number of HIV-seropositive doctors will be seeking such advice in the future.

4.6 What is meant by 'safe sex'?

Essentially, sexual contact with any other animate object is likely to risk possible transmission of infection. Unless the person having sex is alone in a locked room with no windows, it is unlikely that completely safe sex with a 0% risk of them becoming infected will be possible! A better term is 'safer sex'.

There are two approaches to safer sex. Firstly, a reduction in the number of partners so that the risk of encountering a new sexual partner with an infection will be minimized. This is an individual choice and for some will mean no change to their lifestyle whatsoever. Others, however, will have to rethink the type of relationships into which they choose to enter. Secondly, safer sex embodies the concept of indulging in sexual practices which provide satisfaction and enjoyment but which minimize the risk of infection being transmitted. In the context of HIV transmission, sexual practices have thus become divided into three categories: low, medium and high risk. Clearly, the evidence of what is high risk can be most easily gleaned from epidemiological studies of cases in which HIV transmission has occurred. However, it becomes harder to prove that something is of low, or even negligibly low, risk to be called zero risk of passing on an infection. It should also be remembered that when weighing up the risks for transmission of HIV infection, some suggested practices should not be considered low risk for the transmission of other conditions such as pediculosis pubis, syphilis or warts.

The use of condoms has become an important component in the safer sex message. However, it has been clear for a long time that in heterosexual intercourse, condoms do not provide 100% protection against the occurrence of pregnancy. Condoms can be damaged by fingernails, poor storage, improper technique when putting them on and unduly traumatic sexual practices. It has been reported that the rates of condom breakage during anal intercourse are higher than those during vaginal intercourse; therefore, condoms have been produced which are thicker and are more popular amongst gay men and heterosexuals who engage in anal intercourse. Although such propaganda about condoms, as has been provided, has led to the suggestion that using a condom (for any sexual practice) will constitute safer sex, this is erroneous. If a condom breaks during oral sex, the chance that an infection would pass from either of the parties involved to the other, is very much lower than if anal intercourse was occurring between two gay men.

The question then arises that if a new pair of partners who wish to engage in sex use condoms during the initial part of the relationship, how should they proceed if their relationship moves on to a stronger footing and, in the case of heterosexuals, wish to conceive? Many couples are using HIV as a reason for having full check-ups of each other prior to moving their relationship on to a different level. Interestingly, in both heterosexual and homosexual relationships, many couples seem to find heavy petting, i.e. mutual masturbation with or without oral sex, an engaging and fulfilling experience without the need for full penetrative intercourse. Prior to moving their footing on to 'a more stable basis', they often attend genitourinary medicine or other clinics for 'a full check-up'. Such practices and responsibility amongst individuals clearly should be encouraged and made more available.

4.7 Is oral sex safe?

In order to reliably answer this question, it is necessary to identify people who only have engaged in either active or passive oral sexual contact with others, and to assess their seroprevalence rate for HIV infection or for other sexually transmitted diseases. Unfortunately for the epidemiologists, very few such individuals exist. However, it is clear that in surveys of sexual practice in the UK, active oral sexual contact is reported to be engaged in by 80% of heterosexual women and 50% of heterosexual males. Despite this commonly-engaged-in sexual practice by both heterosexual and homosexual couples, there are only two case reports existing where oral sexual contact alone has led to transmission of HIV. One of the cases involved a heterosexual male who had fellatio performed on him without a condom on repeated episodes by a female injecting drug-using masseuse. She was HIV seropositive and passed the infection to him, presumably via this route. The second case was of two gay men, in whom the recipient of the HIV also acquired oral pharyngeal gonorrhoea by engaging in passive oral intercourse without a condom. These cases both add fuel to the advice that condoms should be worn for oral sexual contact which involves putting the penis into the mouth. Ejaculation into the mouth is seen as the most likely route of HIV transmission.

In the case of cunnilingus, the role of the female condom (Femidom) is uncertain at present. It is clear that the major risk to the active partner in this would be if the woman was menstruating. This has been recently highlighted in literature circulated by lesbian organizations to try to minimize the risk of HIV transmission in this group.

4.8 Can HIV infection be transmitted by shaking hands?

No.

5. HIV antibody testing and counselling

5.1 What is pre-test counselling for HIV antibody testing?

The concept of pre-test counselling embodies the principle that the recipient who requests information about the HIV antibody test, either because of a real or imagined perceived risk for acquisition of the infection, will benefit whether their test result becomes positive or negative. If the test result is negative, the individual will have had the opportunity to learn about HIV infection and AIDS, to assess their own past or present risks from infection with HIV and other sexually transmitted diseases, and had a chance to hear about safer sexual practices and general health measures, e.g. stopping smoking, reducing alcohol intake, dietary improvement. If the test result is positive, then the individual will benefit by having been counselled to rehearse the possibility that the result will be positive, to prepare for coming to terms with this result and to have informed access to resources for support and post-test counselling. This latter aspect may involve a continuation of the relationship which was set up in the pre-test counselling session either by doctors, nurses or specific HIV counsellors.

5.2 What should pre-test counselling include?

It should be unhurried, confidential and open-ended. It is vital that the patient does not feel that it is something which has to be endured prior to them passing some imagined hurdle before having a test. It should be portrayed in a positive light by either the doctor or other health professional carrying out the counselling. A simple check list of items to cover is useful, but should not be used to set any agenda or order for items to be gone through. The most important use of this check list is to raise subjects about which the patient can ask their own questions and reach their own conclusions. The pre-test counselling points which do need to be emphasized are:

1. Explanation of what an HIV antibody test is. It needs to be explained

that it is not a test for AIDS, and that special points need to be emphasized in certain cases, e.g. the incubation period of the infection and the window period (i.e. the time between acquisition of infection and seroconversion). It should also be explained how and when the patient will be able to obtain the test result and who will be giving them this result.

2. Risk history. It is vital that a history is taken of sexual behaviour, and any injecting drug behaviour in either the patient or in a sexual partner. History of travel, blood transfusion or the receipt of other blood products should also be taken. By using this history, an individual can weigh up his own risks of being infected by HIV or other infections, but it must be remembered that many patients do not know the risk histories of their sexual partners, and thus may not be able to give the history of their real risk of HIV infection.

3. Confidentiality. It should be made clear that the result is confidential to the staff involved in the care of the patient within the clinic, and that it will not be released to anyone without their explicit consent. The concept of medical confidentiality must be emphasized. It should be clarified whether or not the patient will wish a General Practitioner to be informed of the result and if so, by what means. It is our practise to encourage this.

4. Rehearsal of HIV-positive result. The difference between HIV and AIDS must be emphasized. The medical implications of an HIV-positive result should be outlined, including the need for regular follow-up. The possibility of receiving therapies for HIV infection must be stressed. The clearly defined benefits of AZT and *Pneumocystis carinii* pneumonia (PCP) prophylaxis should be stressed, along with ensuring the patient understands that the time from HIV infection to developing AIDS is on average 10 years. The patient needs to rehearse psychosocial implications of a positive result. Defining who they would tell, how it might affect their employment, housing, family and friends is important.

The issue of life insurance has long been confused. It has recently been clearly re-emphasized by the Association of British Insurers, who represent more than 95% of all British insurance companies, that a person having a negative HIV antibody test will face no discrimination whatsoever because of the act of having that test. If the test is positive, then they have emphasized that all pre-existing life insurance policies will be honoured up to that time, although the patient will no longer be able to take out new life insurance policies. Despite this reassurance, a survey of patients attending a London genitourinary medicine clinic revealed that more than a quarter of those having an HIV antibody test intended to lie about ever being tested in any proposal for life insurance.

5. Transmission of infection should be discussed. In particular, the issue of sexual transmission which would include a detailed discussion of what safer sex means. The use of condoms will be discussed. For men or women who are contemplating becoming parents, it is vital to discuss the risks of transmission via mothers to their children.

6. A general discussion of health promotion usually occurs with a discussion on smoking, alcohol and nutritional lifestyles. If individuals are using other recreational drugs then discussion of this is usually included.

Having done this, some doctors insist on a signed consent for the performance of an HIV test, although the majority do not. In some cases, the patient may decide that after counselling, they prefer to go away and read more literature, think about the issue, and then decide at a later date whether or not to have a test. The majority of people who undergo pre-test counselling do go on to have a test, and it is vital that their information is backed up by written leaflets and booklets.

5.3 How is an HIV antibody test performed?

After counselling and the patient giving their informed consent, a sample of blood is drawn for sending to the laboratory. It is important that the container containing the blood is correctly labelled and accompanied by a test request form signed by a registered medical practitioner. In the interests of confidentiality, some departments utilize patient numbers and dates of birth rather than patients' names on the sample labels and the request forms.

In the laboratory, the serum is separated. The usual test performed for HIV-1 and HIV-2 antibodies is the enzyme-linked immunosorbent assay (ELISA). This is relatively simple and easy to perform. A range of commercial kits are available which enable many samples to be processed simultaneously. In the ELISA, all the viral antigens of HIV are represented and antibodies to any of these may demonstrate a positive result.

It is accepted practise that positive tests and equivocal tests are repeated to confirm their accuracy. This is usually by a different method, and the most widely used alternative to ELISA is Western Blot. The Western Blot method involves electrophoresis of disrupted HIV virions on slab gels. Individual viral antigens are identified.

For both ELISA and Western Blot tests, false positives and false negatives are very rare.

5.4 What should the patient who has had a positive HIV test be told?

At the time of testing for HIV antibodies, an agreement is made with the patient as to when they will receive a result and who will give them their result. This depends on how long the laboratory takes to process the sample and on when the patient finds it convenient to return. The patient should also be asked if they wish anyone to be with them when they are given the result. Some patients prefer to bring a partner, friend or other supportive person with them when they receive a test result. If the result if positive, the patient will obviously be upset. Even patients who expect to have a positive result, because their partners have died from AIDS, will often exhibit a considerable amount of distress at their own seropositivity. It is vital to allow the patient time to come to terms with their result before overloading them with information about measures of immunity, antiretroviral therapies, PCP prophylaxis and clinical trials. Of immediate importance is the patient's psychological as well as physical well-being. However, it does help to set the scene with the patient for what will happen over the next few weeks. Allowing the patient to understand the methods which will be used to determine the stage of their HIV infection, and the significance of tests such as CD4 lymphocyte counts, HIV p24 antigens, and the use of antiretroviral therapies, can allow the patient to see a positive aspect to the management of their illness. At the time of their diagnosis, many patients will 'demand therapy now'. It is important that counsellors try to ensure that the patient takes proper time and consideration over decisions about therapy, and does not rush into the use of treatment without understanding the issues. In cases where this is insisted upon by the patient, it is vital to provide early follow-up to review, and to further explain the situation regarding drugs such as AZT and other antiretroviral therapies.

It is also important in post-test counselling of the HIV-positive patient to discuss relationships — who they will tell about their HIV infection, if anyone. This has often been rehearsed at the pre-test counselling session, but needs to be further reinforced after a positive test result. This will often include discussions about reducing the chances of transmission to others by sexual or other routes.

5.5 What do patients who test HIV negative need in the way of post-test counselling?

The evidence that post-test counselling causes any effect whatsoever in sexual behaviour is lacking, with some studies even suggesting that those who underwent post-test counselling after a negative result had a higher incidence of subsequent sexually transmitted diseases. Despite this, patients who test antibody negative should have clear reinforcement of the information about the transmission routes of HIV, and a firm message that they are not immune from acquiring HIV because they have tested negative.

In patients who have been tested for HIV infection within the 'window period' of an exposure to an HIV-infected source, it is important that post-test counselling sets a new time for a repeat test, and provides continuity of management and support through this. In our current practice, this means having a further test 2 months after the initial episode of exposure.

5.6 Who is a counsellor?

Much has been written about 'counselling' with respect to HIV infection. What is clear is that the issues concerned with gaining the trust and informed consent for a patient to undergo an HIV antibody test exemplify many of the principles which are required for a patient undergoing any invasive procedure and test. The patient should be encouraged to understand the issues and the possible sequelae of either a positive or a negative test. If the physician caring for the patient has the knowledge, time, skill and motivation to achieve this themselves, then they can make a perfectly adequate counsellor. On the other hand, the set-up of many clinical practices means that physicians cannot give unlimited time to patients in order to fulfil this. For another reason, it is often desirable for a patient to see someone separate to the physician who has taken their history, examined them, and possibly dealt with other problems at the same visit. In finding a counsellor who may be a nurse, health advisor, or another trained person in whom to confide about issues which may relate more to social and behavioural factors than those which the patient may view as in the doctor's remit, there is often a value to making such a referral. However, in the end it is the patient's choice whether they simply see a doctor, have the test pros and cons explained to them, agree to have blood drawn and a test performed with the result being given to them by a physician. If the patient chooses this, then it is perfectly adequate. It is every physician's responsibility, however, to ensure that each patient has the opportunity to receive the appropriate counselling, and to give their informed consent prior to undergoing an HIV test. Furthermore, it is their responsibility to ensure that the HIV test is placed in context of an approach designed to prevent HIV transmission, and to promote the concept of sexual and behavioural health in their patients.

6. Early HIV infection

6.1 What is the incubation period of HIV infection?

The acute illness associated with seroconversion seen with HIV infection usually occurs 2–6 weeks after exposure. Occasionally seroconversion occurs later, between 3 weeks and 3 months after infection. Although for practical purposes it is reasonable to assume that an individual who is negative 3 months after the last exposure to HIV will remain so, seroconversion is theoretically possible up to a year. Cases such as this have been recorded, although often they are not well documented, and other more recent sources of infection have not always been rigorously excluded.

6.2 What is seroconversion?

The term seroconversion in association with HIV infection refers to the time at which antibodies against the virus become detectable in the peripheral blood.

6.3 What are the features of the seroconversion illness?

The acute infection or seroconversion illness seen in association with HIV exposure is like glandular fever. Typical features include fevers, a rash, myalgias, arthralgias, malaise, lymphadenopathy, sore throat, gastrointestinal symptoms, headache and photophobia. The illness is usually of acute onset and generally lasts between about 3 and 14 days.

The rash is generally maculopapular occurring mainly on the trunk and limbs. It can be associated with a diffuse enanthema of the oral cavity and stomatitis. Occasionally large oesophageal ulcers occur and diarrhoea is common.

Occasionally neurological symptoms are seen at the time of the seroconversion illness. These include an acute reversible encephalopathy with disorientation, loss of memory and consciousness. Acute meningitis, myelopathy and neuropathy have also been described.

There can be a marked lymphopenia and associated immunological impairment at the time of the acute HIV infection. Consequently, some of the opportunistic infections associated with later HIV infection, such as oesophageal candidiasis and *Pneumocystis carinii* pneumonia (PCP), may rarely be seen.

6.4 Does everyone who contracts HIV infection experience this seroconversion illness?

It is unusual for people who contract HIV infection to present at the time of seroconversion, unless some of the more serious manifestations occur. Usually these illnesses are diagnosed in retrospect, when the patient with HIV infection presents for other reasons and history reveals a particularly severe isolated illness episode some years previously. However, only about 30% of people are able to identify a possible seroconversion illness, and it is probable that a relatively high proportion of people have a sub-clinical acute infection with the virus.

6.5 In a patient who presents with symptoms of fever, sweats, lethargy, malaise, pharyngitis and headache, what clinical factors can be used to differentiate EBV mononucleosis from primary HIV infection?

Primary HIV infection is more commonly associated with a sudden onset, little or no tonsillar hypertrophy and enanthema on the hard palate alone. In contrast, EBV mononucleosis usually has a slower onset and is character-ized by a marked tonsillar hypertrophy and enanthema on the border of the hard and soft palate. Exudative pharyngitis is common in EBV disease and not in primary HIV infection, whereas oral ulcers are much more common in primary HIV infection. A skin rash, usually maculopapular and non-specific on the trunk and neck, is rare unless antibiotics are given in the case of mononucleosis, but is common in primary HIV infection. In addition to mononucleosis, the differential diagnosis of primary HIV infection should include CMV mononucleosis, toxoplasmosis, rubella, viral hepatitis, secondary syphilis, disseminated gonococcal infection, herpes simplex virus infection, other viral infections, drug reactions and dermatological conditions.

6.6 What investigations should be performed if a seroconversion due to HIV is suspected?

As previously stated, HIV antibodies are not usually detectable at the time of acute HIV infection. It is sometimes possible to detect HIV antigen in the blood of patients with acute HIV infection, and techniques such as the polymerase chain reaction (PCR) may become useful as their accuracy is better defined. Unless a dual infection was present, the Paul Bunnell test would be negative. It is, however, impossible to definitively differentiate acute HIV infection from other causes of glandular fever in most cases. If suspected, the patient should have serial HIV antibody tests over the next 3–6 months.

It is mandatory to perform syphilis serology on patients who are sexually active with non-specific symptoms including skin rashes and/or oral ulceration.

6.7 What happens after the acute infection?

There usually follows a latency period when the patient is completely asymptomatic and there is no clinical evidence of HIV infection.

6.8 Is it true some people with HIV infection are asymptomatic for a long time?

Yes, most people who contract HIV infection appear to have an asymptomatic period of years rather than months. As HIV infection has only been recognized as a disease entity relatively recently, and as the course of the illness can be long, it is impossible to say what the maximum length of this asymptomatic phase can be, and whether everyone who contracts the infection will necessarily progress to symptomatic disease and death.

The longest outcome study presently published on a group of patients known as the San Francisco Cohort, has found that about 63% of patients have developed an AIDS diagnosis after a follow-up time of approximately 12 years. Of the remainder, a relatively small number of people have symptomatic HIV infection, and approximately 30% remain asymptomatic after 12 years follow-up.

6.9 Do asymptomatic HIV-antibody-positive people need any special advice to help keep them well?

As with most other chronic conditions it has not been proven that changes in lifestyle help to prolong patients' good health. However, if a patient requests advice, it would seem sensible empirically to give similar advice about healthy living to general health promotion. This also has the added advantage of helping the patient feel that they have some control over their illness. Measures usefully undertaken could include improved nutrition, reduction in tobacco and alcohol intake, stress reduction, stopping or reducing recreational drug usage and safer sex, which will not only help to prevent the spread of the illness, but might also avoid any further damage to the immune system as a result of repeated antigenic stimulation.

6.10 What about any treatments?

There is now research evidence to suggest that AZT delays progression to symptomatic HIV infection in asymptomatic patients with laboratory evidence of immunosuppression. Such treatment is licensed for use by those with evidence of impairment of the immune system demonstrated by a reduced CD4 lymphocyte count. Clinical trials of AZT and combinations of antiretroviral therapy are in progress. For a more complete discussion on this please refer to Chapter 14.

6.11 Do any special measures need to be taken when managing incidental illness in the HIV patient?

In the asymptomatic patient, incidental illnesses should be managed in the same way as in the HIV-negative patient.

In the symptomatic patient, incidental illness needs to be differentiated from complications of HIV infection. Also, in some instances it might be necessary to alter management to compensate for immune impairment; for example, possibly having a lower threshold to prescribing antibiotics in respiratory infections, and when prescribing to give reasonably high doses and adequate courses.

In the patient with late-stage HIV infection, it is also necessary to take into account the prognosis from the HIV infection when considering the management of incidental chronic illnesses. Meeting the patients needs and wishes are of paramount importance in such cases.

6.12 Is it safe to vaccinate a patient with HIV infection?

This depends on the proposed vaccination. The basic rule is to be careful with live vaccines. BCG is the only vaccine that is absolutely contraindicated. Patients should be warned that if they are given the conventional oral polio vaccine (Sabin) which is a live vaccine, they may excrete the virus for a protracted period. Consequently, all likely contacts should be vaccinated at the same time, or it may be preferable to give the killed injectable (Salk) formulation. Opinions differ about giving yellow fever vaccination. It is probably reasonable to give it to the asymptomatic and relatively immune competent patient, but it may be advisable to seek expert advice in each individual case. All other vaccinations can safely be performed at any stage of the disease. They are best given as early in the course of the disease as possible, as immunological response will be best. It is advisable to check the hepatitis B status of all patients with HIV infection and vaccinate if necessary.

Recently, some workers have demonstrated an increase in HIV plasma viraemia after certain vaccinations. Further work will be needed to define whether vaccines may result in disease progression. Until then, the individual risk of acquiring the infection must be weighed against this hypothetical risk.

6.13 What is persistent generalized lymphadenopathy (PGL)?

PGL is defined as enlarged lymph nodes of at least 1 cm in diameter in two or more extra-inguinal sites, that persist for at least 3 months in the absence of any current illness or medication known to cause enlarged nodes.

The nodes are usually symmetrically affected, and the groups most often enlarged are in the posterior and anterior cervical chains, axillary and submandibular regions. The nodes are usually soft, mobile, not fixed to the skin and non-tender.

6.14 What is the significance of PGL?

PGL was described before HIV was isolated, when it was noticed that there were a group of patients presenting with enlarged lymph nodes, often from the then recognized risk group for AIDS, some of whom later went on to develop signs, symptoms and opportunistic infections of AIDS-related complex and AIDS itself.

The presence of PGL in the patient with HIV infection certainly doesn't appear to be associated with a worsening of prognosis. It has been suggested that the presence of enlarged lymph nodes is actually a good prognostic sign indicating an active immune system. It has also been suggested that the sudden loss of enlarged lymph nodes may immediately precede progression of the disease. Both these claims are hard to substantiate.

6.15 What should be checked for when assessing the patient with early HIV infection?

The main thrust of the history and examination should be aimed at detecting the presence of any signs and symptoms associated with the late-stage HIV infection. For further details of this see Chapters 7 and 8. However, particular attention should be paid to signs and symptoms of general ill health, and to examination of the skin, oral cavity and possibly central nervous system (see Table 6.1).

The most useful investigation in early HIV infection is estimation of the CD4 lymphocyte count. The frequency of measurement depends upon the stage of disease. In patients with CD4 lymphocyte counts well above the normal range (500 cells mm^3), annual investigation is appropriate. In patients whose counts are only just above the normal range, more frequent investigation is necessary in case the patient wishes to consider

Table 6.1   Check list in HIV infection (this should be adapted depending on the disease status of the patient)

General	Sweats and rigors
	Weight loss
	Lymphadenopathy
	General well-being
Skin	Dry skin
	Seborrhoeic dermatitis
	Psoriasis
	Folliculitis
	Herpes simplex
	Herpes zoster
	Kaposi's sarcoma
Respiratory system	Cough
	Dyspnoea
Mouth	Gingivitis
	Oral candidiasis
	Oral hairy leucoplakia
	Kaposi's sarcoma
Gastrointestinal tract	Diarrhoea
	Dysphagia
	Pain
	Peri-anal disease
Central nervous system	Mood
	Concentration
	Memory
	Peripheral neuropathy
	Motor weakness
	Retinopathy

Table 6.2   Useful baseline investigations in the patient with HIV infection

Haematology	Full blood count
	Lymphocyte subsets
Biochemistry	Urea and electrolytes
	Liver function tests
Microbiology	HIV antibody
	HIV p24 antigen
	Hepatitis B serology
	Syphilis serology
	Cryptococcal antigen
	Toxoplasma antibody titre
	Cytomegalovirus antibody titre
Radiology	Chest X-ray

early antiretroviral treatment. The relevance of this investigation is discussed in Chapters 3 and 14.

At the time of initial presentation, a full history and examination to detect any incidental disease should be performed. The clinician should be particularly aware that as HIV is most usually a sexually transmitted disease, other sexually transmitted diseases often coexist.

It is useful to perform a series of baseline investigations at the time of first presentation which may aid interpreting investigations in the symptomatic patient (see Table 6.2).

6.16 When an HIV-antibody-positive patient with no previous symptoms attends a doctor for a routine checkup, which particular clinical features should be searched for?

As in standard medical practice, it is vital to take a good history. Early features of HIV-associated diseases manifest most often in the mouth or on the skin. In more severely immunosuppressed patients, it is vital to search for symptoms of conditions which may affect visual fields (CMV retinitis), cause dyspnoea, cough and fever (PCP), result in headaches, fits (toxoplasma cerebral abscess) and gastrointestinal manifestations, such as diarrhoea (cryptosporidiosis) or dysphagia (CMV oesophagitis). These examples indicate the wide range of symptoms which can occur in patients at different stages of HIV-related disease. The particular conditions which occur at particular stages of immunosuppression can often be highlighted with prior knowledge of the patient's most recent CD4 lymphocyte count and a previous history of any pre-existent conditions indicating the degree of immunosuppression which HIV has caused in that particular patient.

On clinical examination, it must be emphasized that there may well be nothing to find. It is not unusual to find an HIV-infected patient with no symptoms and with no positive finding on full physical examination. This usually indicates that the patient will have a correspondingly high CD4 lymphocyte count. Signs often associated with a moderate degree of immunosuppression (CD4 lymphocyte counts of 200–400 cells/mm^3) are the presence of extra-inguinal lymphadenopathy, seborrhoeic dermatitis especially on the face, oral candidiasis or oral hairy leucoplakia in the mouth, and other skin problems such as eczema, recurrent herpetic infection, molluscum contagiosum and condylomata acuminata. In addition, it is important to weigh the patient and form a general assessment of their nutritional status.

As patients are unable to examine visually the whole of their skin surface, it is vital for even asymptomatic patients to be examined thoroughly to search for lesions of Kaposi's sarcoma, or other skin conditions which may be out of the individual patient's visual field. This also applies to lesions on the soles of the feet and the backs of the thighs and buttocks.

In a patient who is asymptomatic and has no clinical findings on examination, it is usual practice to perform a 3–6-monthly check of haemoglobin, white cell count and platelets, CD4 lymphocyte count, and other locally accepted markers of immunosuppression and disease progression. These are discussed in Chapter 3.

6.17 Should a patient with normal cell immunity and no evidence of clinical immunosuppression but who is HIV antibody seropositive have regular check-ups for other sexually transmitted diseases?

Clearly the answer to this question depends on taking an accurate history of the patient's sexual behaviour. Patients who have not engaged in any sexual contact over the past 2 months and who are asymptomatic need not be submitted to a local genital examination. In taking this history however, it is important to recognize that many patients may say 'no' to the question, 'have you had sex?', when they mean 'yes' to the question, 'have you had safer sex?' Some patients will not call sex 'proper' unless penetrative activity has occurred. It is important to recognize that sexually transmitted conditions can be passed on during safer sexual practices. Examples of this include scabies and pediculosis pubis, pharyngeal gonorrhoea during oral sex, and even a recent case of gonococcal ophthalmia, when a patient during safer sex had a partner (with gonorrhoea) ejaculate into his eye! Thus, assuming an accurate history has been taken to define a risk of acquiring a sexually transmitted condition, or the patient complains of symptoms suggestive of a sexually transmitted condition, then a standard sexually transmitted disease examination with microbiological testing should be carried out. This will include a local test taken for gonococcal and chlamydial infections, as well as serum tests for syphilis and hepatitis B.

HIV-antibody patients who acquire sexually transmitted diseases should be treated in exactly the same way as patients who are HIV negative or of sero-status unknown. However, certain conditions, particularly chronic viral warts and genital herpes, may be more severe and recalcitrant to treatment because of the underlying immunodeficiency in the HIV-seropositive patient who acquires them. Similarly, cases of syphilis in patients who are HIV seropositive need to be treated with regimens of antitreponemal drugs which have adequate penetration into the cerebrospinal fluid.

Despite counselling about safer sexual techniques and more often than not the patient's enthusiasm to participate in these, many patients will suffer lapses of their good practice in maintaining safer sexual techniques. It is vital that clinicians and others seeing HIV-seropositive patients continue to remind patients in a non-judgemental way about safer sexual techniques. Positive continued reinforcement of such measures may help to prevent some of the lapses, which is not only beneficial to the patient in avoidance of acquiring sexually transmitted diseases, but also decreases the risk of passing HIV on to a sexual partner.

7. AIDS related complex (ARC)

7.1 What is ARC?

ARC is the term used for the stage of HIV infection which is characterized by two or more of the constitutional signs and symptoms of HIV infection listed in Table 7.1, in the absence of a super added AIDS-diagnosing condition. As with all other stages of HIV infection, it represents a largely artificial diagnostic category, that was introduced before HIV was discovered and antibody testing became available. At that time, it was noted that there was a group of patients in whom a collection of fairly non-specific signs and symptoms were commonly seen, and these patients frequently went on to develop one of the AIDS-diagnosing conditions. It is now widely accepted that HIV is best seen as a disease continuum, characterized by gradually deteriorating immune function. The conditions discussed in this chapter become increasingly prevalent, as the number of CD4 lymphocytes, and hence immune competence, decreases. The term ARC is still widely used by people with HIV infection and has some use in classification.

Lymphadenopathy has already been discussed in Chapter 6, and the presence of this sign in conjunction with any of the other conditions listed in Table 7.1 will give an ARC diagnosis.

7.2 Is there any treatment available for the night sweats and fatigue?

The night sweats and fatigue are both symptoms that result from the chronic infection that HIV causes. Their severity varies very much from patient to patient, some people suffering from a bit of lethargy and a night sweat every 2 weeks or so, while others feel completely washed-out and experience nightly sweats. The tendency is for the symptoms to increase in severity with decreasing immune function and hence increasing viral load.

Anti-pyretics, such as paracetamol and aspirin taken at night, can be useful in people with mild to moderate sweats. For people with more

Table 7.1   Constitutional signs and symptoms of HIV infection seen in ARC

Lymphadenopathy	
Night sweats	
Fatigue	
Weight loss (less than 10% of body weight with no underlying cause)	
Diarrhoea (with no demonstrable underlying cause)	
ENT problems	Chronic sinusitis
	Post nasal drip
Oral cavity problems	Oral candidiasis
	Oral hairy leucoplakia
	Gingivitis
	Aphthous ulceration
Skin problems	Seborrhoeic dermatitis
	Tinea infections
	Folliculitis
	Impetigo
	Herpes simplex
	Molluscum contagiosum
	Viral warts
	Psoriasis
	Xeroderma
Thrombocytopenia	

severe sweats or associated marked fatigue, AZT or another antiretroviral agent can produce symptomatic relief. However, relief is not universal, but if the patient is much disabled by these symptoms it is reasonable to offer antiretroviral therapy.

In late-stage HIV infection, generally after AIDS has been diagnosed, fatigue can severely limit the patient's quality of life. In such cases, amphetamines have been tried, but success has been limited.

7.3 What about the weight loss?

Weight loss in HIV can be due to the general catabolic effects of chronic infection, and the more specific effects of acute episodes, such as an opportunistic infection, anorexia and diarrhoea with associated malabsorption.

The first line of attack is generally dietary advice to suggest how to maximize calorific intake, given either by a specialist dietician or the patient's clinician. Specific high calorie supplements, such as build-up drinks, can be a useful adjunct to this advice.

Various steroid hormones with anabolic effects, such as testosterone or methyl progestogen, have been extensively tried in an attempt to promote weight gain or at least to reduce weight loss. Controlled trials of these drugs have been disappointing unless they are given in such high doses that side-effects often outweigh the benefits. This is especially true of methyl progestogen, which commonly causes erectile impotence in men.

7.4 How should diarrhoea be managed in the patient with HIV infection?

The main thrust of management of diarrhoea in the HIV-infected patient is to attempt to isolate any of the pathogens that are commonly responsible for causing diarrhoea in the context of HIV infection. A full history should be taken to establish duration and volume of diarrhoea. Investigations should include repeated stool cultures (most experts would recommend at least three stool cultures and possibly up to six), sigmoidoscopy and biopsy, blood cultures, and possibly upper gastrointestinal endoscopy with jejunal biopsy via a crosby capsule.

Organisms which present more frequently in the HIV-infected patient as a cause of diarrhoea include *Giardia lamblia*, *Entamoeba histolytica*, salmonella species, shigella species, campylobacter, cytomegalovirus (CMV), *Cryptosporidium muris*, *Microsporidium* and *Mycobacterium avium-intracellulare* (MAI). Salmonella, CMV, *Cryptosporidium*, *Microsporidium* and MAI are all discussed in Chapter 8.

Amoebiasis and giardiasis are both commonly seen in the HIV-infected patient. They can generally be diagnosed by direct microscopy or fresh stool specimens. They should be treated with conventional therapy, that is, the relevant dose of metronidazole. Relapse is common, and repeat stool specimens should be sent after treatment has been completed.

Campylobacter and shigella infections are diagnosed by stool culture. The best therapeutic agent for shigella is usually found by sensitivity testing. Nearly all cases of campylobacter will respond to erythromycin. Approximately one-third of the cases of diarrhoea seen in patients with HIV infection will not yield an obvious pathogen. There are two possible explanations for this. Firstly, it is well demonstrated that HIV itself attacks the lining of the gut causing an enteropathy. Secondly, there is always the possibility of an undiagnosed occult pathogen. In these cases, symptomatic treatment should be embarked upon using conventional opiate-based anti-diarrhoeals, which in severe cases may possibly include slow-release morphine tablets. Whilst continuing with symptomatic treatment, further investigations should be performed, which will often reveal a treatable pathogen at a later date.

7.5 What ENT problems occur in patients with HIV infection and how should they be managed?

Chronic sinusitis and post-nasal drip are both commonly seen in patients with HIV infection. Their high incidence is thought to be a result of the generalized decrease in cilial function seen in association with HIV infection. Topical steroid preparations, such as dexarhinaspray and aerosolized beclomethasone have been used with good effect to produce symptomatic relief. Nasal decongestants have yielded poor results. Acute exacerbations often require systemic antibiotics. Various surgical procedures, such as sinus lavage, have been tried in patients who are very severely affected, but results have been disappointing.

7.6 What pathology can be seen in the mouth?

Conditions which are commonly seen in the mouth of patients with symptomatic HIV infection are oral candidiasis, oral hairy leucoplakia (OHL), gingivitis and aphthous ulceration.

7.7 How should oral candidiasis be managed?

It is worth mentioning that oral candidiasis is relatively rare in young people in the general population, unless there is a history or recent antibiotic therapy. It is very common in association with HIV infection, and its presence in an otherwise fit and healthy young person should raise suspicion of HIV infection.

Most cases of oral candidiasis will respond rapidly to topical antifungal agents, such as nystatin drops/lozenges or amphotericin lozenges. Some patients try to avoid the ingestion of pharmaceutical agents, and in such cases, live yoghurt or acidophilis may provide relief.

If the condition fails to respond to the above agents, a short course of systemic antifungal agents, such as ketoconazole, itraconazole or fluconazole, will produce a quick cure.

7.8 Is prophylactic treatment against recurrent oral candidiasis necessary?

Up until recently, there was a vogue for giving patients with recurrent oral candidiasis long-term prophylactic treatment with one of the systemic antifungal agents. This has been shown to have two major disadvantages. Firstly, the high cost of such treatment and secondly, the development of multi-resistant strains of Candida. It would now generally be advised that patients who suffer from frequent recurrences of oral thrush should be given a supply of either topical or systemic antifungal agents to be taken for a few days when symptoms recur.

Various methods which may help to reduce the frequency of relapse include decreasing sugar intake in the diet, ingestion of live yoghurt, and use of chlorhexidine mouthwashes and acidophilis tablets which are freely available in most health food shops.

7.9 What is oral hairy leucoplakia (OHL)?

OHL most usually presents as white corrugated plaques seen on the side of the tongue. It can, however, occur anywhere in the oral cavity and has also occasionally been found to involve the oesophagus. It is easy to differentiate from Candida as the plaques are adherent, unlike Candida, which can readily be scraped off with a wooden spatula.

It appears to be caused by the Epstein–Barr virus as this has been found in biopsy material. OHL appears to be unique to HIV infection, and its discovery on routine examination should be considered diagnostic of the condition. It is not uncommon for patients to present with HIV infection following their dentist noticing patches of OHL.

7.10 How should OHL be managed?

OHL is certainly not a pre-malignant condition. The lesions are painless and therefore it presents a largely cosmetic problem. Plaques frequently spontaneously resolve.

If a patient finds that OHL poses unacceptable cosmetic problems, acyclovir in a dose of 800 mg 4 times a day usually resolves the condition. Unfortunately, it tends to recur quickly on cessation of treatment. It is, therefore, generally best to reassure the patient that OHL is inconsequential and to encourage them to ignore it.

7.11 How should gingivitis be managed?

Gum infections and dental abscesses are very common in association with HIV infection, and as ever in medicine, prevention is better than cure. Patients with HIV infection should be advised to have regular dental check-ups and to maintain good dental hygiene. Useful advice for this includes careful brushing, the use of dental floss, and perhaps the use of antiseptic mouthwashes such as chlorhexidine.

If gingivitis does occur, it will usually respond well to antibiotic therapy, such as penicillin V 500 mg 4 times a day, or metronidazole 400 mg 3 times a day. Supplementary dental advice should be sought as an adjunct to antibiotic therapy.

7.12 What should I do for a patient who has persistent aphthous ulceration?

It is certainly true that severe aphthous ulceration, sometimes even extending into the oesophagus, can be a problem for patients with HIV infection. If the ulcers are only mild, benzocaine lozenges can be a useful analgesic. Topical steroids, such as hydrocortisone lozenges or betamethasone pellets, can help to reduce inflammation and pain and accelerate resolution.

If the ulcers do not respond to these measures, it should be noted that both CMV and herpes simplex infections can cause ulcers on the lips or inside the oral cavity. Patients should be referred for appropriate culture or biopsy. If no infective cause can be found, thalidomide and systemic steroids have both proved useful in cases of resistant painful oral and oesophageal ulcers.

The use of oral bandages (e.g. Orahesive) has been reported to provide relief of symptoms and permit improved oral intake in patients with severe aphthous ulceration. These may also be useful in patients with ulcerated oral Kaposi's sarcoma (KS).

7.13 What skin problems might I encounter in a patient with HIV infection?

As would be expected in patients with a depressed cellular immunity, viral and fungal skin infections are very common. These include herpes simplex, herpes zoster, molluscum contagiosum, seborrhoeic dermatitis, tinea infections and folliculitis, which can be either fungal or bacterial in aetiology. The bacterial infections, impetigo and cellulitis, are also commonly encountered.

There may also be an increase in skin conditions of unknown aetiology, such as psoriasis and xeroderma. KS, which constitutes an AIDS diagnosis, is also frequently seen. This is discussed in Chapter 9.

7.14 How should the patient with frequently recurrent herpes simplex be managed?

As most cases of HIV infection are sexually transmitted, it is not surprising that there is a parallel increase in the incidence of herpes simplex infection, be it oral, genital or peri-anal. As immune function is depressed, relapses tend to occur more and more frequently. It is therefore not unusual to find patients who suffer with frequent painful attacks of herpes simplex in any one of the three sites mentioned above. It should also be noted that episodes tend to run a more protracted course.

Patients with an active relapse should be managed conventionally with acyclovir at a dose of 200 mg 5 times a day for 5 days. Patients who have repeated episodes of herpes simplex infection, or particularly severe recurrences, may wish to consider prophylactic oral acyclovir in an attempt to suppress relapses. The best method is to start with a dose of 400 mg twice daily and to titrate this down until the minimum inhibitory dose is established, which may be as little as 200 mg per day. Topical acyclovir is of little value in either treating attacks or preventing relapse.

7.15 Is there anything unusual about herpes zoster in patients with HIV infection?

Episodes of shingles in young people are relatively unusual, and it is one of the conditions which should raise a suspicion of HIV infection. This is especially true if an attack of shingles affects more than one dermatome, which is rare in the immunocompetent patient. It is also possible to see people who have a past history of chickenpox suffer from another bout or develop coexistent shingles and chickenpox.

The course of shingles in the HIV-infected patient tends to be more protracted, and post-herpetic pain and scarring are more frequently encountered. Therefore, it is advised that people with HIV infection should be treated with oral acyclovir at a dose of 800 mg 5 times a day for 1 week. If the ophthalmic division of the trigeminal nerve is involved, then intravenous acyclovir is indicated. Obviously, management should include adequate analgesia and soothing topical agents, such as calamine lotion.

7.16 How should warts and molluscum be managed?

Warts and molluscum are both commonly seen in people with HIV infection. As a result of deficient cell-mediated immunity, they tend to be widespread, and it is rarely possible to eradicate them. Therapy is aimed at trying to limit their extent for cosmetic purposes. This is best achieved by cryotherapy with liquid nitrogen, which is unlikely to result in significant scarring.

7.17 What is the treatment of seborrhoeic dermatitis?

Seborrhoeic dermatitis is exceptionally common in patients with HIV infection, to a degree that the vast majority of patients are likely to be affected at some time during the course of their illness. It also tends to be more extensive than is typically seen, possibly involving the arms and even the legs. It is speculated that the pityrosporum yeast is important in the aetiology of the condition, causing a chronic inflammatory reaction.

This speculation is supported by the fact that the condition responds well to topical combinations of steroids and antifungal agents. The most popular of these are either Daktacort^R or Canesten HC^R. In resisting cases, Trimovate^R is useful.

7.18 How should other skin infections be approached?

Although some of the other skin infections which have already been listed are seen with increased frequency and possibly increased severity in people with HIV infection, treatment is along conventional lines.

Tinea infections should be treated with conventional topical antifungals, such as miconazole or clotrimazole. Folliculitis can be either fungal or bacterial in origin and should be treated as appropriate, although sometimes topical steroids are necessary to provide complete resolution.

Impetigo, which is of staphylococcal origin is best treated with oral flucoxacillin, and cellulitis being streptococcal in origin is best treated with systemic penicillin V.

7.19 Why is psoriasis included in the list of ARC conditions?

Psoriasis is another common condition in the general population, and has an increased incidence and severity in association with HIV infection. The exact reason for this is unknown, but it is obviously associated with the impairment of cell-mediated immunity. It is very common for people to develop psoriasis for the first time after becoming HIV positive, and those people with pre-existing psoriasis often notice a marked increase in severity of the condition.

The principles of management are as in the patient without HIV infection using the same wide range of treatments.

7.20 What causes thrombocytopenia and how should it be managed?

There can be many causes for a generalized pancytopenia in patients with HIV infection, including bone marrow suppression secondary to drugs, such as sulphonamides, ganciclovir and AZT, the direct bone marrow suppressive effects of HIV itself, and involvement of the bone marrow in infective or malignant processes, such as MAI infection or lymphoma. In these cases, it should be managed by removing or treating the underlying cause.

A more selective and specific thrombocytopenia is sometimes also seen. This is autoimmune in aetiology, and is the result of the generation of a specific antiplatelet antibody as part of the disease process of HIV infection. This can lead to very low platelet counts and, occasionally, spontaneous bruising and bleeding is seen.

Obviously many cases are multi-factorial in origin, and even if an autoimmune-type thrombocytopenia is suspected, it is important to avoid the use of bone marrow suppressive drugs, and to treat any possible infection that may involve the bone marrow.

The autoimmune-type thrombocytopenia can be quite difficult to manage. Steroids have been of limited value, and obviously there are great concerns about their use causing further suppression of an already impaired immune system. If the patient is not already on AZT therapy, commencing this can produce marked rises in the platelet count. In severe cases, when platelet counts drop very low or there is spontaneous bleeding, platelet transfusion is probably the best management. Splenectomy has been tried with good results in some patients. However, trials have failed to conclusively prove its benefit.

8. AIDS — opportunistic infections

8.1 When can the patient with HIV infection be said to have developed AIDS?

The onset of AIDS is specified as the time of diagnosis of one of the list of AIDS-defining conditions; these are the major opportunistic infections and malignancies (Kaposi's sarcoma (KS), non-Hodgkin's lymphoma and primary cerebral lymphoma), neurological manifestations, and profound weight loss seen in association with HIV infection (see Table 8.1).

Table 8.1 AIDS-diagnosing conditions

1. Major opportunistic infections
2. Malignancies Kaposi's sarcoma
   Non-Hodgkin's lymphoma
   Primary cerebral lymphoma
3. Loss of greater than 10% body weight with no demonstrable cause
4. HIV encephalopathy
5. Possibly in the future, CD4 lymphocyte count less than 200 cells/mm³

As with the other stages of HIV infection already discussed, an AIDS diagnosis is a largely arbitrary point in the clinical continuum of HIV infection. This is underlined by the fact that the AIDS-diagnosing conditions take no account of the underlying function of the immune system. It would be difficult to say that someone who has made a complete recovery from *Pneumocystis carinii* pneumonia (PCP) has a worse prognosis than someone who is asymptomatic but with laboratory evidence of very severe immune impairment. With this in mind, there have been recent moves to include a CD4 lymphocyte count of less than 200 cells/mm³ in the criteria for diagnosing AIDS. At the time of writing, this potential development has not occurred, but it may well do so in the future.

The malignancies seen in AIDS and the neurological manifestations of AIDS will be discussed in Chapters 9 and 10.

8.2 What is an opportunistic infection?

An opportunistic infection is one which takes advantage of impairment in the host's immune responses to produce a particular clinical and pathological picture. It can be caused by an organism which is not normally pathogenic in man, or an organism which causes a disease process that is increased in severity or duration in the immune-impaired host. Thus many of the infections already described in Chapter 7 can be considered to be acting opportunistically in the HIV-infected patient. Similarly, opportunistic infections may occur in patients with other causes of immune impairment, such as the iatrogenically immunocompromised post-transplant patient.

For the purposes of this chapter, the term opportunistic infection will be used to describe the major AIDS-defining opportunistic infections seen in association with HIV infection.

8.3 What are the main opportunistic infections?

Over 50 opportunistic infections are included in the American Centers for Disease Control classification of AIDS. The vast majority of these are rarely encountered in clinical practice. Opportunistic infections may be caused by bacteria, viruses, fungi and protozoa. The organisms producing important opportunistic infections in HIV infection are shown in Table 8.2.

Opportunistic infections can be organ-specific or disseminated. The individual infections will be discussed by body system as much as possible and the systemic infections will be discussed at the end of this chapter.

8.4 Which patients with HIV infection are susceptible to opportunistic infections?

The opportunistic infections PCP and oesophageal candidiasis have both been described in patients experiencing a seroconversion illness. Opportunistic infections have been described at all subsequent temporal stages of the disease. However, it is rare to see opportunistic infections in patients without laboratory evidence of severe immunological impairment. As a general rule of thumb, it is possible to say that opportunistic infections are very rare in patients with CD4 lymphocyte counts greater than 200 cells/mm^3, and unusual in patients with CD4 lymphocyte counts greater than 150 cells/mm^3. The more the immune system deteriorates, the more the patient becomes susceptible to opportunistic infections. Some infections such as *Mycobacterium avium-intracellulare* (MAI) complex and cytomegalovirus (CMV) retinitis are rare except in very late-stage HIV infection, and are usually seen in patients who have already had at least one AIDS-diagnosing condition.

Table 8.2 Important opportunistic infections seen in AIDS

	Organism	Site affected/ clinical process
Viruses	Cytomegalovirus	Lung Central nervous system Gut Disseminated
	Herpes simplex	Lung Central nervous system Gut Disseminated
	Papovavirus	Central nervous system
Bacteria	*Mycobacterium* (*tuberculosis, avium-intracellulare* complex)	Lung Central nervous system Gut Disseminated
	Salmonella	Gut Disseminated
Fungi	*Pneumocystis carinii* (now thought to be fungal rather than protozoal)	Lung Disseminated
	Cryptococcus	Lung Central nervous system
	Candida	Gut Central nervous system
Protozoa	Toxoplasma	Central nervous system Disseminated
	Cryptosporidium	Gut
	Microsporidia	Gut

8.5 Which opportunistic infections affect the lungs?

Disorders of the respiratory system are very common in HIV infection. A list of organisms which cause pulmonary infections in AIDS is given in Table 8.3.

PCP is the most common opportunistic infection seen in association with HIV infection. CMV is frequently isolated in HIV-associated pneumonias, but its clinical significance is dubious (see below).

MAI, which may be isolated from the sputum usually as part of a disseminated infection, is discussed later in this chapter. Pulmonary infection with *Mycobacterium tuberculosis* (MTB) does not constitute an AIDS diagnosis unless the infection is spread outside the lungs and lymph nodes. This, along with *Cryptococcus neoformans* and *Toxoplasma*

Table 8.3   Organisms causing pulmonary infections in AIDS

Pneumocystis carinii
Cytomegalovirus
Mycobacterium avium-intracellulare
Mycobacterium tuberculosis
Cryptococcus neoformans
Toxoplasma gondii
Histoplasma capsulatum
Nocardia asteroides
Pyogenic bacteria

gondii, both of which usually affect other systems, will also be discussed later in this chapter.

Histoplasma capsulatum and *Nocardia asteroides* are both rare causes of respiratory disease in AIDS patients.

Bacterial pneumonias account for approximately 10% of chest infections seen with HIV. Diagnosis is made by routine sputum and blood culture and they are treated as a non-HIV patient would be.

8.6 How does PCP present?

PCP is by far the most common opportunistic infection seen in association with HIV infection. Before the widespread use of specific primary prophylaxis against the condition (see below), it accounted for some 60% of new AIDS diagnoses, either alone or in tandem with KS. Although the use of primary prophylaxis has decreased the frequency and severity of episodes of PCP, it is still estimated that up to 80% of AIDS patients will suffer an attack at some time during their illness. It should also be stressed that the pneumonia is often recurrent, and so it is essential that all clinicians are familiar with the presenting signs and symptoms of this condition. It is not uncommon for patients with HIV infection to present for the first time with a severe full-blown episode of PCP.

The classification of the organism *P. carinii* has caused much argument, but most people would now accept that it is a fungi rather than a protozoa. It has been recognized as causing opportunistic infections since the early 1900s. It was seen in epidemics in the orphanages of Eastern Europe in the post-war years. Following this, it was rarely seen until its association with HIV infection in the early 1980s. *P. carinii* can cause infection in several organs, but it is very rare outside the lungs.

The patient presenting with PCP classically gives a history of insidious onset of lethargy, shortness of breath, cough and mild pyrexia, which increase gradually in severity over a period of weeks or possibly even months. The shortness of breath is initially only seen on exertion, but progresses to affect the patient at rest. The cough is usually non-productive, unless there is a coexistent bacterial pneumonia (see below) or the patient is a heavy smoker. The patient's temperature tends to be less than 38°C.

Examination is often remarkably unhelpful in diagnosing PCP. In more severe cases the patient will look unwell and will be short of breath at rest. The chest is frequently clinically clear unless there is a coexistent bacterial pneumonia.

If suspected PCP is the first presentation of possible HIV infection, it is useful to look for other possible signs of the condition, such as oral candidiasis, oral hairy leucoplakia, seborrhoeic dermatitis or weight loss.

8.7 How can we differentiate PCP from a bacterial chest infection or another pneumonia?

As stated above, PCP tends to be fairly insidious in onset. The presence of a purulent production associated with the cough or any marked chest signs, would suggest a bacterial pathogen as the cause, as would a temperature above 38°C. The patient with PCP may appear to be disproportionately short of breath.

However, to make a definitive diagnosis of PCP requires investigation (see below) and, as previously stated, bacterial chest infections can often coexist with PCP. A patient with a productive cough in whom PCP cannot be excluded and who does not appear unwell enough to warrant immediate hospital referral, is best managed by starting on an antibiotic that will not interfere with the clinical course of PCP, such as erythromycin or amoxycillin. The patient should be reviewed 48 hours later, by which time it should be evident if there has been no improvement, and then be referred for further investigation.

8.8 What special investigations support or confirm a provisional diagnosis of PCP?

The initial changes seen on chest X-ray with PCP are the presence of a perihilar haze, which in more severe cases will progress to diffuse homogenous infiltrates, mainly in the mid and upper zones with peripheral sparing. Patchy consolidation is more likely to suggest a bacterial chest infection. It is not however possible to rule out PCP on chest X-ray changes alone.

Blood gas estimation will usually, but not always, demonstrate a hypoxia, but again this is a non-specific finding.

Exercise oximetry almost always shows desaturation of capillary oxygenation in response to exercise. This will give a raised suspicion of PCP.

The definitive diagnosis is by direct demonstration of the presence of *P. carinii*, either through an induced sputum (using nebulized saline in an attempt to get samples from the alveoli where pneumocysts are in greatest concentration), or bronchoscopy with bronchio-alveolar lavage if sputum induction fails. Trans-bronchial biopsy is now rarely used because of the high incidence of morbidity and mortality associated with this procedure.

If all the above investigations fail to produce a definitive diagnosis but the clinical picture is very suggestive of PCP, the patient should be treated as presumptive PCP with a full course of relevant therapy.

8.9 How should PCP be treated?

The treatment of PCP depends to some extent on the severity of the attack as gauged by blood gas estimation.

A mild attack (patient relatively undistressed by symptoms and blood oxygen of greater than 10 kPa) can be managed with oral therapy, and treatment is now often undertaken as an outpatient. The two most common regimens are either co-trimoxazole 480 mg 8 tablets twice daily, or clindamycin 600 mg 4 times daily in combination with primaquine at a dose of 15–30 mg once a day.

A moderately severe attack of PCP (arterial oxygen between 8 and 10 kPa) definitely requires hospitalization because of the risk of deterioration. Co-trimoxazole can be used at the same dose intravenously, transferring to oral therapy once the patient is stable, or clindamycin and primaquine in combination can be used either orally or intravenously.

Severe PCP (arterial oxygen less than 8 kPa) should definitely be treated with intravenous therapy. It is now almost unanimously suggested that steroids should be used in such cases, and their use leads to a significantly decreased mortality. There are wide variations in the recommended steroid regimen.

Many other agents have been used in the therapy of PCP, of which pentamidine is most widespread. It still represents a very useful second-line therapy, and is first given intravenously, and then in a nebulized form concurrent with the intravenous therapy, the latter being halted once the patient is stable.

The duration of therapy for all regimens is generally 3 weeks. However, some patients with mild attacks can cease therapy after 14 days.

Piped oxygen should be used as necessary for moderate and severe cases.

8.10 What are the common side-effects seen in treatment?

Some degree of nausea and vomiting is the most common side-effect seen with co-trimoxazole, and this is almost universal when it is given orally in high dose. About one-third of patients have to cease therapy because of drug rashes, and fever is also common. Less common side-effects include leucopenia, thrombocytopenia and abnormal liver function tests.

Early studies of clindamycin and primaquine suggested that drug rashes were very frequent. However, more recent studies suggest that only about 1 in 10 patients develop a hypersensitivity reaction.

8.11 Is recurrence common?

Yes! It is almost inevitable that anyone who has experienced an attack of PCP will sooner or later suffer with another episode, unless they are given post-treatment prophylaxis. Prophylactic regimens should be the same as for those people receiving primary prophylaxis, that is, co-trimoxazole 960 mg twice daily 3 times per week, dapsone 100 mg once daily, or nebulized pentamidine 300 mg once a fortnight.

8.12 When is MTB an AIDS diagnosis?

MTB is considered an AIDS diagnosis when it occurs outside the lungs and outside the lymph nodes. Its incidence is generally much increased in association with HIV infection, especially in people who have contracted the condition in Africa or who have a history of intravenous drug use. Non-disseminated pulmonary tuberculosis is considered an ARC diagnosis.

8.13 How should MTB be managed in the AIDS patient?

Treatment is essentially the same as for any other patient group using a standard triple-therapy regimen. There is differing opinion as to whether courses of treatment should be more protracted than in the non-HIV patient, and some clinicians would recommend life-long prophylaxis with a single agent, most usually isoniazid.

8.14 How does oesophageal candidiasis present and how should it be treated?

Oesophageal candidiasis presents classically with dysphagia and retrosternal pain. The presence of oral candidiasis and particularly pharyngeal plaques would be supportive of the diagnosis. A definitive diagnosis can be made with upper gastrointestinal endoscopy (which will show the classic white plaques in the oesophagus) and culture of biopsy material.

Systemic antifungal agents are essential for successful management of the condition, and the drugs used would either be ketoconazole 200 mg twice daily, itraconazole 200 mg once daily, or fluconazole in a dose between 50 and 200 mg once daily. The growing trend is towards short sharp courses of systemic antifungals of about 5 days, or as long as is necessary to produce cessation of symptoms. The patient can then be given a supply of the antifungal agent and advised to restart therapy if a symptomatic relapse occurs.

8.15 What conditions can CMV cause in the gastrointestinal tract?

CMV can cause infection of the gastrointestinal tract anywhere between the oral cavity and the anus, including the biliary tract. It most commonly presents as ulcers, and by far the most common sites are in the oesophagus or the colon.

CMV oesophagitis causes similar symptoms to oesophageal candidiasis, that is, retrosternal pain and dysphagia. It is diagnosed at upper gastrointestinal endoscopy either at the time of investigation of these symptoms, or if systemic antifungals fail to give relief. A typical punched out ulcer will be seen, and biopsies will reveal the typical histological appearances of CMV infection.

CMV colitis causes diarrhoea associated with blood, pus and mucus. In fulminant cases it can lead to perforation and peritonitis, and will almost inevitably be fatal. It is diagnosed by biopsy at either sigmoidoscopy or colonoscopy, which will again show the typical histological features of CMV infection. Early diagnostic suspicion is vital to the management of this condition.

The treatment of CMV infection will be discussed in the section on CMV retinitis later in this chapter.

8.16 What problems does cryptosporidium infection cause?

The parasite *Cryptosporidium muris* generally causes infection of the surface mucosa of the gastrointestinal tract. It can also sometimes affect the bile duct, pancreatic duct and gallbladder. When affecting the gut, it causes gradual fusion of the villi and consequently a malabsorbative-type diarrhoea.

In the non-immunocompromised patient, cryptosporidial diarrhoea occurs in episodic outbreaks and cases are self-limiting. In the context of the severely immunocompromised patient with HIV, infection poses a much greater threat. Owing to the patient's inability to clear the infection, there can be a gradual increase in malabsorption leading to increased quantities of diarrhoea. In the most severely affected patients, this can mean up to 8 litres of watery diarrhoea per day.

Many different agents have been used to attempt eradication of cryptosporidium from the gut once it is present. However, so far it would be difficult to claim that any one of these is successful. It is therefore essential to try to prevent patients contracting the condition. Cryptosporidium is a commensal of most domestic water supplies, and patients with HIV infection and moderate to severe immune impairment should be advised to boil all their water before drinking. Advice on commercial mineral waters is difficult, as frequently it is unknown whether or not they contain cryptosporidium.

8.17 What are the common opportunistic infections seen in the central nervous system (CNS)?

CMV can cause infection of the retina, and also encephalitis and polyradiculopathy. The last two are relatively uncommon. The encephalitis is often seen as a confusional state associated with disseminated CMV infection, and the polyradiculopathy causing a progressive spastic paralysis. They both respond poorly to treatment.

Toxoplasmosis can cause cerebral abscesses and consequently present as any other space-occupying lesion, and the fungus *Cryptococcus neoformans* can lead to meningitis and also cause abscesses in the brain.

Progressive multifocal leucoencephalopathy is thought to be caused by the papovavirus. Diagnosis is suggested by neurological imaging and, if appropriate, confirmed by brain biopsy. There is no effective therapy.

8.18 How does CMV retinitis present?

CMV retinitis classically presents as gradual visual blurring and field loss. It should however be suspected in anyone with late-stage HIV infection who has a visual disturbance. It is very unusual to see the condition in people who have not had a pre-existing AIDS diagnosis or with a CD4 lymphocyte count of above 100 cells/mm^3. Other characteristic symptoms include seeing floaters and partial or complete loss of visual fields.

Presumptive diagnosis rests on seeing characteristic retinal changes of soft exudates and retinal haemorrhages. These are sometimes seen in people who do not complain of any visual symptoms, but the patient should still be treated as if they have CMV retinitis.

It should be noted that the vast majority of clinicians working in the HIV field would look to ophthalmological colleagues to confirm the diagnosis, and from a pragmatic point of view, the non-expert should refer any patient with visual disturbances for urgent ophthalmological opinion. This is because CMV causes a progressive and irreversible destruction of the retina.

8.19 How should CMV infections be treated?

It will by now be obvious that CMV can cause infections in many different systems in the AIDS patient. It can also cause generalized infection. Unfortunately, the only two agents available to treat CMV infection have to be given intravenously. They are ganciclovir (DHPG) and Foscarnet (Phosphonoformate). Ganciclovir should be given at a dose of 5 mg/kg twice daily intravenously. The duration of treatment is generally 3 weeks. However, 14 days is sometimes adequate for CMV oesophagitis or colitis.

The major side-effect of ganciclovir is bone marrow suppression leading to neutropenia, thrombocytopenia and anaemia. The risk of these haematological side-effects is greatly increased if the patient is receiving AZT and this should be discontinued during acute therapy.

The dose of Foscarnet is calculated according to body weight and serum creatinine. The major side-effect of Foscarnet is nephrotoxicity and the risk of this can be greatly reduced by oral prehydration (getting the patient to drink between 1 and 2 litres of fluid orally before treatment is commenced). Another relatively common side-effect of Foscarnet therapy is the development of mucosal ulcers which are thought to be caused by direct toxicity from contact with the drug. These are most commonly seen on the penis and the risk of them decreases if the urine is weak and also if the penis is washed after micturition. They can also occasionally be seen in the mouth.

8.20 Is prophylaxis necessary to prevent reactivation of CMV infection?

Relapse of CMV infection is common at any site. If the affected site is the colon or the oesophagus, it is relatively easy to give another course of treatment and spontaneous healing will occur. Unfortunately, as CMV retinitis causes irreversible destruction of the retina, any degree of reactivation of the infection leads to a significant risk of blindness. Therefore, patients who have experienced an episode of CMV retinitis are advised to have maintenance treatment with either ganciclovir or Foscarnet to prevent relapse. As previously stated, both these drugs are only effective when given intravenously. Consequently, patients with CMV retinitis are advised to have an in-dwelling intravenous catheter inserted through which maintenance therapy can be delivered.

Both ganciclovir and Foscarnet are given in half their treatment doses once a day 5 days a week to prevent relapse. However, this is obviously the cause of great inconvenience to the patient. Additionally, all the associated risks of having a long-term in-dwelling catheter, most notably septicaemia, should be remembered. Recent research has shown that where a district nurse is available to supervise therapy, the risk of septicaemia is greatly reduced with a parallel increased survival.

8.21 What are the signs and symptoms of cerebral toxoplasmosis?

Cerebral infection with toxoplasmosis leads to the formation of abscesses. Consequently the signs and symptoms are the same as for any other space-occupying lesion. These are severe headaches, confusion and focal neurological signs, often associated with seizures developing over a period of 1–2 weeks.

Toxoplasmosis can also cause infections at other sites in the body in the AIDS patient, but these are relatively rare.

8.22 How should toxoplasmosis be investigated and treated?

The single most useful investigation for suspected cerebral toxoplasmosis is computed tomography (CT) of the brain. This classically shows solitary or multiple ring-enhancing lesions often with surround oedema. Toxoplasma serology is unreliable in diagnosing acute CNS infection, as many patients have previously been exposed and have positive toxoplasma antibodies. However, a rising titre would suggest reactivation.

Definitive diagnosis requires demonstration of the parasite in biopsy brain tissue, but this is rarely carried out because of the associated morbidity and mortality and, if strongly suspected, patients are treated presumptively.

Toxoplasma infection is treated either with Fansidar tablets in high doses, in conjunction with folinic acid to prevent severe bone marrow suppression, or with a combination of clindamycin and pyremethamine, also in conjunction with folinic acid. The second regimen is gaining favour because of the risk of Stevens–Johnson syndrome associated with Fansidar.

Patients who develop seizures as a result of toxoplasma infection require anticonvulsants which can sometimes be discontinued once the infection is controlled. Also, patients with a severe attack often benefit from dexamethasone which helps to decrease cerebral oedema.

Despite the severe-sounding nature of toxoplasmosis affecting the brain, the prognosis is actually remarkably good and most patients affected can expect to achieve an almost full recovery and live for at least a year.

8.23 How does cryptococcal meningitis present and how should it be managed?

Patients with cryptococcal meningitis often suffer with prodromal symptoms of fatigue, fever and weight loss. As the illness evolves a headache develops and this may sometimes be associated with nausea, vomiting and photophobia. Neck stiffness occurs in the majority of patients but is not universal. Occasionally, focal neurological signs may develop.

The diagnosis is usually made by Indian ink staining and culture of cerebrospinal fluid (CSF) for the organism *Cryptococcus neoformans*. Measurements of cryptococcal antigen in CSF and serum is also useful.

The treatment of cryptococcal meningitis in AIDS involves using the standard therapy of intravenous amphotericin B either alone or in combination with flucytosine. A 6-week course of this treatment will usually produce eradication of the organism from the CSF. Relapse, however, is common and lifelong maintenance with oral fluconazole at a dose of 400 mg a day is recommended to try to reduce the frequency of this.

8.24 What is progressive multifocal leucoencephalopathy (PML) and how is it managed?

PML is the consequence of CNS infection with papovavirus in AIDS patients. The clinical features are very variable and can range from limb weakness to visual loss or a rapid deterioration in mental state. Patients usually deteriorate rapidly over a period of weeks and months, becoming more and more encephalopathic and debilitated until their death.

Diagnosis is with CT or magnetic resonance imaging (MRI) of the brain which demonstrate hypodense, non-enhancing white matter lesions. Diagnosis would be confirmed by brain biopsy, but this is rarely performed because of the poor prognosis of the condition and the associated morbidity and mortality.

Many different agents have been tried to treat the condition, but so far no therapy has altered the clinical course.

8.25 We have discussed organ-specific opportunistic infections, but which can be disseminated?

As already alluded to earlier in the chapter, many of the organisms which are responsible for opportunistic infections can cause disseminated disease. This is particularly true of toxoplasmosis which can affect many different systems and also produce a disseminated infection.

The infections which are almost inevitably disseminated are the *Mycobacterium avium-intracellulare* (MAI) complex and leishmaniasis. Leishmaniasis generally presents as a pyrexia of unknown origin associated with weight loss and anaemia. It is diagnosed by culture of the organism, histological examination of liver biopsy and bone marrow, or splenic aspiration. It is relatively uncommon in the UK but is seen with greater prevalence in people who have travelled in the Americas, Africa or continental Europe. It is treated with a protracted course of either stibogluconate or pentamidine intravenously. Relapse is common and weekly maintenance with intravenous pentamidine is recommended to try to decrease the frequency of this.

8.26 What is MAI complex infection and how does it present?

MAI is also known as atypical mycobacterium. The organism is ubiquitous in the environment and rarely causes a pathological picture in the immunocompetent patient. It is very commonly found in the HIV-infected patient with late-stage disease, and can affect almost any system in the body. It most commonly causes disseminated disease.

The classical presentation is, as with leishmaniasis, a pyrexia of unknown origin associated with anaemia and weight loss. Variations on this depend on whether any one particular system is predominantly affected and include diarrhoea if the organism is present in large quantities in the gastrointestinal tract, and shortness of breath if it is widespread in the lungs.

8.27 How is MAI diagnosed and treated?

Diagnosis is based on acid fast staining or culture of stool, blood or tissue specimens. Liver biopsy samples give a high rate of isolation by direct acid fast staining.

Treatment is difficult as MAI is highly resistant to most of the conventional antibiotics used in mycobacterium infections. Many different agents have been tried with varying success. Most commonly a triple-therapy regimen is employed and drugs used include rifabutin, clofazamine, ciprofloxacin, cycloserine, amikacin and many other agents. Response is measured by a decrease in transfusional requirements, decrease in pyrexia and increase in weight.

8.28 When is herpes simplex an AIDS-defining illness?

Herpes simplex is considered an AIDS-defining illness when one crop of ulcers lasts for greater than a month without resolution. If a correct diagnosis is made, therapy with acyclovir should be able to prevent this occurring.

8.29 What is the prognosis for someone who has developed an opportunistic infection?

The prognosis for opportunistic infections is very variable depending on the individual infection and severity of the episode. It is commonly believed that developing an AIDS diagnosis indicates a very rapid death, but this is far from true. The best prognosis is probably associated with an episode of PCP, with a life expectancy after a first episode of 3 years. Oesophageal candidiasis and cerebral toxoplasmosis also carry a very good prognosis with a life expectancy of well over a year. Conversely, CMV retinitis infection carries an average prognosis of about 7 months and MAI infection gives an even worse outlook. It is however important to encourage the HIV patient who has had an opportunistic infection diagnosed to recognize that they may well still have much good quality life left.

8.30 How is AIDS defined on weight loss?

A loss of greater than 10% of ideal body weight and the absence of any underlying demonstrable cause are criteria for an AIDS diagnosis. This is obviously a very difficult criteria to satisfy as many of the infections and malignancies associated with AIDS can be quite elusive to diagnosis and can obviously cause profound weight loss.

It is also true to say that some degree of wasting is almost universal in people who have severely symptomatic HIV infection.

9. HIV and malignant disease

9.1 How does HIV infection result in development of malignant disease?

The development of neoplastic disease as a complication of immuno-deficiency is a phenomenon which was well described before the advent of the HIV epidemic. For instance, patients receiving iatrogenic immunosuppressive therapy for renal transplantation had been shown to have an increased instance of malignant tumours, particularly lymphoma, which occurred 35 times more commonly in this group. Similarly, in patients with primary cell-mediated immunodeficiencies, the risk of developing malignant disease is 10 000 times that of an age-matched control population. Interestingly, in children born with defects of antibody production, there is no such increase in neoplasia; instead, the major sequela is an increased incidence of bacterial infections.

The mechanism for the development of these opportunistic tumours in patients with immunosuppression seems to be due to the failure of specific T lymphocytes to maintain immunosurveillance for the recognition and deletion of malignant cell clones. It appears that HIV infection results in an increased occurrence of certain tumours via such a mechanism of immunosuppression, rather than directly due to HIV infection.

9.2 What type of malignancies occur in patients with HIV infection?

One of the initial diseases which led to the description of AIDS as a specific syndrome was Kaposi's sarcoma (KS). At present the aetiology of this condition remains unclear and the therapeutic options available remain limited. Originally, more than 50% of homosexual men presenting with AIDS had KS, although this figure has now fallen to under 20%. The other AIDS-defining malignancy is non-Hodgkin's lymphoma. This is seen in about 5% of patients with AIDS and these tumours are all of the B-cell phenotype.

Other conditions which have been described in patients with AIDS,

Table 9.1   Malignancies in HIV infection

AIDS defining	Non-AIDS defining
Kaposi's sarcoma	Hodgkins disease
B-cell lymphoma	Squamous carcinoma
	Malignant melanoma
	Plasmacytoma
	Small cell carcinoma of the lung
	Germ cell testicular tumour
	Seminoma
	Adenocarcinoma of the colon

but which may not be causally related to HIV infection or immunosuppression are shown in Table 9.1.

9.3 What is KS?

KS is a multifocal proliferative disorder which is generally regarded as neoplastic but which has several unique characteristics. It was originally described by the Hungarian dermatologist Moritz Kaposi in 1872. Three different types of patient appear to develop this condition. The classical form of the disease tends to occur in middle-aged to elderly males, with a higher incidence being seen in certain Jewish, East-European or Mediterranean populations. Secondly, in African patients, endemic KS is particularly common in sub-Saharan regions. This condition includes an aggressive and disseminated form of KS. The third type of KS is seen in association with immunosuppression. This may be in patients receiving immunosuppressive medications, or in patients with HIV infection and AIDS. In patients with HIV infection, KS primarily affects homosexual or bisexual men, but it rarely occurs in drug users or recipients of blood products. This observation has led to speculation that the cause of KS is a sexually transmitted agent which is most common in homosexual or bisexual men. Despite extensive research, there is no proof that hepatitis B, syphilis, cytomegalovirus, herpes simplex, or Epstein–Barr virus infections are the cause of KS.

9.4 How is KS diagnosed?

Many patients who develop KS are themselves the first to notice the skin lesions. However, as early small lesions of KS may occur in sites out of sight of the patient, it is essential that clinicians regularly perform full mucocutaneous examinations of their HIV-infected patients. The first sign of a cutaneous lesion of KS is usually a macular erythematous lesion only a few millimetres in diameter. Over the following 1–2 weeks this discoloured area often becomes infiltrated and raised, and the lesion will darken to take on a reddish purple hue. Smaller tumours are painless and usually asymptomatic except for cosmetic disturbances. The tumours vary in size, number and distribution, with some individuals having a solitary lesion whilst others develop tens, or even hundreds, within a matter of weeks or months. Lesions on the neck and trunk are usually elongated and often follow the natural skin cleavage lines. Lesions are often symmetrical. Involvement of the mouth is common with about one-third of patients having oral lesions at the time of their initial diagnosis of cutaneous KS. Despite these typical clinical features, it is vital that a diagnostic biopsy be performed. This is important because other conditions can mimic KS (e.g. benign naevi, cat scratch lesions, Molluscum contagiosum), and because the confirmation of this AIDS-defining condition may influence the patient's decision to opt for particular types of therapy. The histology of a typical nodular KS lesion consists of proliferations of spindle cells in the dermis which entrap red blood cells. In the surrounding dermis blood pigment deposition is common with patchy, associated, chronic inflammatory cell infiltrates rich in plasma cells. The histological appearances of earlier disease are more subtle, and it is vital that the pathologist is alerted to the possibility of KS as a diagnosis to aid their examination of the biopsy.

The diagnosis of non-cutaneous KS may be problematic, but will usually be based on the localized appearance of symptoms. In the case of pulmonary and pleural involvement by KS, the development of chest symptoms along with a bloody pleural effusion and nodular appearances on chest X-rays are highly suggestive of KS. Gastrointestinal bleeding or signs of obstruction may be related to the development of KS in the upper or lower gastrointestinal tract. Diagnosis by endoscopy and biopsy in such situations is the most usual form of investigation.

9.5 Does AZT affect KS in patients with HIV infection?

Yes. It appears that up to one-third of patients with KS will undergo partial resolution of lesions upon starting AZT. However, this is rarely total and further progression of disease tends to occur after a period of 6–12 months. Whether or not the use of AZT therapy in patients with HIV infection but without KS will prevent the development of this skin condition is unknown.

9.6 What treatments are available for HIV patients with KS?

Firstly, it must be said that treatment is not appropriate for every patient with KS. Many patients prefer to avoid the need for drug or other therapies and are comfortable with using makeup and other cosmetic measures to cover up any visible KS lesions. As neither the underlying HIV infection nor the associated immunosuppressive disorder can be completely reversed, the primary goal of therapy for KS at present has to be palliation. If cosmesis alone is unacceptable to patients, or they are developing pain, oedema or other symptoms from their KS, then alternative forms of therapy are available. These may be divided into local and systemic therapies.

9.7 What local therapies are available for the treatment of KS?

Local cryotherapy using liquid nitrogen has been successfully used for small (< 1 cm diameter) KS lesions. The use of intralesional chemotherapy using Vinblastine injected into the base of a lesion will often promote shrinkage and fading of the lesion. However, this can often result in a hyper-pigmented area after treatment. The mainstay of local therapy for KS is radiotherapy, although this is less appropriate for people with widespread disease. It is particularly useful in cases of lymphatic obstruction, especially when this involves the face. Intra-oral and pharyngeal lesions can be treated with radiotherapy but a severe mucositis has been observed with high frequency following this treatment.

9.8 What systemic therapies are available for people with HIV infection and KS?

The problem of using cytotoxic drugs for the treatment of systemic disseminated KS is the furtherance of immunosuppression in HIV patients. Although there may be some remission of KS, the likelihood of the development of opportunistic infections needs to be weighed against the use of systemic immunosuppressive therapy. Vincristine and Bleomycin have been used in patients with HIV-associated KS because each is subjectively well tolerated and the incidence of serious toxicity is low. Unfortunately, the cumulative toxicities of each of these drugs necessitate administration on an alternating basis. Etoposide is also active in KS; however, the frequency of alopecia makes it a poor choice for patients who are primarily being treated for cosmetic purposes. Adriamycin may be the most useful active single agent in AIDS-associated KS. Current research is looking at combination therapy, particularly involving interferons. Alpha-interferon has been shown to have antiproliferative and anti-HIV activity. However, in patients who are primarily being treated to try to enable them to improve their quality of life, the side-effects of interferon treatment appear to cause considerable disturbance. Thus, quality of life of patients under therapy has to be properly evaluated and show benefit for the treatment to have widespread usage.

9.9 If a patient presents with a small solitary lesion, should it be treated?

Yes. As a solitary lesion will require a biopsy for confirmation of the diagnosis, it is usual to perform an excision biopsy which will be both curative and diagnostic.

9.10 In a patient with four cutaneous lesions of KS, three on the trunk and one on the face, should these lesions be treated?

That is up to the patient. It is clear that local treatment of KS lesions has no impact on the development of others. KS is not a metastasizing cancer. AZT therapy should be offered if the patient is not already receiving it. A discussion should take place with the patient about the range of therapies available, both local and systemic. The patient may opt for treatment of certain lesions but not others. This depends on the sites of the lesions and the patient's lifestyle. Whilst some patients are particularly concerned about lesions which might be visible when they are wearing swimming costumes, others might be much more concerned about a lesion in their mouth. It is up to the individual physician and their patient to decide on which lesions should be treated and which should not. Whether the patient opts for treatment or not, it is vital to provide suitable psychological support, and to make available cosmetic services for the patient if required.

9.11 If a patient with previously asymptomatic HIV infection develops symptoms and signs of gastritis and even haematemesis, is this likely to be due to GI-associated KS in the absence of visible lesions?

No. In general, patients with visceral KS have lesions present on the skin or in the oral cavity. It is highly unlikely that an otherwise asymptomatic patient would develop severe KS in the stomach or oesophagus without the presence of KS elsewhere. Knowing the CD4 lymphocyte count could also have a bearing on this. Visceral or disseminated KS is unusual in patients with CD4 lymphocyte counts in the normal range. As with all HIV patients who develop symptoms and signs, an investigation for non-HIV-related causes has to be run parallel with investigations for HIV-associated diseases.

9.12 What are non-Hodgkins lymphomas (NHLs)?

NHLs are a heterogenous group of malignancies. Their biological behaviour can range from highly aggressive malignancies, with few long-term survivors, to indolent tumours, requiring no therapy. Approximately

70% of NHLs are of B-cell origin, 20% are derived from T lymphocytes and 10% from mixed origins. The first cases of NHLs in homosexual men were reported in 1982, and increasing numbers have been reported since that time. The finding of an intermediate- or high-grade B-cell NHL in an HIV-infected individual constitutes an AIDS diagnosis. Commonly, advanced extranodal disease is found at presentation and median survival times have been short.

9.13 How do NHLs present in HIV patients?

Commonly the presentation is of a patient with widespread disease involving multiple extranodal sites at the time of diagnosis. In 42% of these patients, central nervous system (CNS) disease occurs and in 33% the bone marrow is involved. Other sites of disease include the rectum, heart and pericardium, and common bile ducts. Some cases of NHLs in HIV-infected patients are confined to the CNS. The most common presenting symptoms are confusion, lethargy and memory loss. Rarely, patients may also present with hemiparesis, aphasia, cranial nerve palsies, headache or seizures.

9.14 Do women with HIV infection have an increased chance of developing cervical cancer?

Studies of the prevalence of abnormal cervical cytology in women with HIV infection have suggested that they have an increased risk of developing cervical intraepithelial neoplasia compared with non-HIV-infected women. However, it is important to exclude confounding variables before accepting this data. Women who may have acquired HIV infection heterosexually may also have been at risk of other sexually transmitted diseases, including those which promote the development of cervical neoplasia. Controlled studies have now begun to delineate a relationship between the development of premalignant disease of the cervix and HIV infection. It is increasingly clear that it is the level of immunosuppression which primarily determines the woman's risk of developing cervical neoplasia. There have been reports of an increase in cervical invasive cancers amongst some women with AIDS, but the relationship between HIV and the development of cervical neoplasia awaits further delineation.

9.15 Should patients with HIV infection who are receiving cancer chemotherapy receive AZT?

It is clearly beneficial that patients with HIV infection and AIDS continue to receive an antiretroviral therapy. The advantages and disadvantages of continuing such therapy need to be weighed up for each individual patient. In general, the toxicity of AZT and cytotoxic agents on the bone marrow often provides a cumulatively excessive myelosuppressive effect resulting in pancytopenia. Increasing use of the antiretroviral ddI may permit the continuation of an antiretroviral without the myelosuppressive effects of AZT. Furthermore the use of specific colony stimulating factors (e.g. granulocyte colony stimulating factor) may enable patients to tolerate considerable myelosuppressive therapies without developing clinically significant problems.

10. Psychiatric problems in patients with HIV infection

10.1 What are the most common psychiatric presentations in patients with HIV infection?

HIV infection is associated with psychiatric morbidity in a number of ways. Firstly, there is the chance coincidence of HIV occurring in a patient with a previous psychiatric history or a predisposition to develop a psychiatric illness. Secondly, there are the psychosocial factors associated with having HIV infection, which are also linked with psychiatric morbidity, for example, a diagnosis of a fatal illness, multiple bereavements or loss of physical functioning. Thirdly, there are mechanisms by which HIV infection may indirectly cause organic brain syndromes, via secondary infections leading to acute organic brain syndromes, or have a primary effect leading to a chronic brain syndrome.

The most common psychiatric presentation is that of adjustment disorder. This is a time-limited exaggeration of a normal response to a stressful event, such as diagnosis of HIV infection, first AIDS-related illness or first dramatic weight loss. Adjustment disorders may take the form of excessive anxiety, low mood, alcohol abuse or a mixture of behaviours. However, unlike the more severe psychiatric syndromes, they resolve within weeks. Counselling is an important intervention and may prevent a worsening of the patient's mental state.

Affective disorders become more common as illness progresses, and have been found by some researchers to be particularly prevalent during the AIDS related complex (ARC) stage of the illness, when patients have a very unclear prognosis, with much uncertainty and loss of control over their bodies. Affective disorders are characterized by a disturbance of mood with inappropriate depression or elation, and are usually accompanied by abnormalities in thinking and perception arising out of the mood disturbance. During depression, patients feel that they are particularly unworthy and that they have very little of value and, at its extreme, they feel life is not worth living. The mood in major depressive illness is persistently low and is qualitatively different from normal unhappiness. There is a loss of reactivity to certain circumstances. There can be a diurnal rhythm, with mood being worse on awakening and improving towards the evening. The mood is pervasive, regardless of circumstances. There is a decreased tempo, a reduction in the quantity of speech, guilt, self-blame, worthlessness and hypochondriasis, with impaired concentration or slowed thinking, as well as an indecisiveness which is not associated with incoherence. There may also be suicidal, morbid and paranoid ideations. These are the important signs, as the somatic signs of poor appetite, weight loss, insomnia, loss of energy and fatigue are likely to be strongly affected by the presence of HIV and are therefore not such good indicators of depression.

Alcohol and substance abuse can start or be aggravated by the stresses associated with HIV infection. Some patients binge on alcohol for long periods of time as a form of denial of their condition. Poor nutrition, with dramatic weight loss and neurological signs can sometimes be due to alcohol and vitamin B deficiency rather than HIV infection.

Personality disorders may be present in a small percentage of HIV-infected patients and will present a challenge for the carers, as the patient's general difficulties in relating to other people will be reflected in their relationships with their doctors. Careful networking with other involved agencies will be necessary to provide support, boundaries, and appropriate medical and psychiatric care.

Psychosis of a manic type occurs in a small percentage of patients with HIV infection. This usually occurs in those with symptomatic AIDS, although the mania may appear in patients with a psychogenic psychosis precipitated by particular stress.

Acute and chronic organic brain syndromes do occur in HIV-infected patients who have severe end-stage illness; these patients are not seen so commonly in the community or by psychiatrists but are mainly dealt with by hospital physicians. Secondary infections associated with immune suppression can cause acute brain syndromes, and HIV itself can cause chronic organic brain syndromes in a small percentage of patients at the end stage of their illness.

10.2 Is there anything special about bereavement in patients with HIV illness, and what distinguishes a normal bereavement reaction from an abnormal bereavement reaction?

Patients with HIV infection can sometimes be exposed to multiple bereavements. This may be because of the nature of HIV transmission, for example, sexual transmission within a close group of friends or acquaintances, or shared needles in a small community of drug users. Sometimes the patient has insufficient capacity to work through the bereavements without some help from a professional agency. The nature of HIV transmission can also complicate bereavement, with the patient feeling guilt or shame in addition to the loss.

Uncomplicated bereavement or typical grief is characterized as follows: there is a stunned phase where emotions are blunted, lasting from a few hours to 2 weeks. This is followed by a mourning phase, in which there is intense yearning and distress. There is great anxiety, with emotions of unhappiness, futility, symptoms of anorexia, restlessness and irritability. At the same time, there is a preoccupation with the deceased and there may be transient hallucinatory episodes, for example, hearing the dead person speak. This is accompanied by either guilt or denial. The final phase is acceptance and readjustment which can occur several weeks after the onset of the mourning. The duration of typical grief varies in different cultures. On average, it lasts 6 months but may continue for a year.

Atypical grief is characterized as follows: firstly, it is chronic lasting longer than the 6 months or 1 year mentioned above. A typical depressive illness may emerge, with morbid preoccupation accompanied by worthlessness, prolonged functional impairment and marked psychomotor retardation. Other features include excessive guilt, denial, identification with the dead person and antisocial behaviour. An alternative atypical grief might be that of inhibited or delayed grief, for example, a patient who appears to have no response at all to the death of a close friend but who, some months later, begins to go through the usual process of bereavement and perhaps has difficulty in linking the two experiences. Thirdly, there are non-specific and mixed reactions which indicate atypical grief, for example, a stress-induced psychosis, or the start of a neurotic syndrome such as panic disorder.

It appears to be important for patients to ritualize their grieving to some extent, for example, to be encouraged to visit the grave of the dead person, and to arrange to set aside time in which to think about the deceased. Often there is some idealization of the deceased to start with, and patients may feel shocked by the anger against the deceased which will follow.

10.3 How should depression be treated in patients with HIV infection?

The treatment for depression in patients with HIV infection should be the same as that in the general population. The primary psychosocial interventions firstly include social manipulations such as supporting re-housing, family support, and general counselling, with hospital admission where there is suicide risk, resistance to outpatient treatment, self-neglect or severe retardation. Various psychological therapies can be applied, for example, dynamic psychotherapy (which helps the patient to understand their present difficulties in terms of their past relationships and their current relationship with the therapist) or cognitive therapy (where treatment is aimed at challenging cognitive errors such as generalization and automatic thoughts in individuals who are over-interpreting their world in critical self-defeating styles). Antidepressants should be used in patients with somatic symptoms of depression. The maximum dosage should be maintained for 3–4 weeks before full benefit can be seen, and therapy should be continued for 6–12 months after recovery from the depression. HIV patients are noted to be more sensitive to side-effects, both anticholinergic and parkinsonian, and therefore it may be that new antidepressants need to be used which have fewer anticholinergic side-effects.

10.4 How should patients with alcohol dependency syndrome and HIV infection be managed?

Alcohol dependency is common in the populations at risk from HIV infection. Individuals dealing with the stress of progressive illness may well increase an existing alcohol habit, or may begin to use alcohol to deal with the stress or even to mask a depression. In contrast to this, the impact of an HIV diagnosis and the implications of prognosis can motivate some patients into receiving treatment for alcohol problems. The alcohol can mimic some signs and symptoms of HIV infection, such as weight loss and neuropathy, and will aggravate poor absorption of nutrients. The critical clinical issue is whether the individual should alter his or her alcohol consumption and, if so, whether that individual can any longer exert control over his or her alcohol ingestion. Alcoholics are those excessive drinkers whose dependence on alcohol has attained such a degree that it shows noticeable disturbance or interference with their bodily and mental functions, their personal relationships and economic functioning, or who show prodromal signs of such a development, in which case they require treatment. There should usually be evidence of either tolerance or withdrawal symptoms, as well as patterns of alcohol ingestion associated with impaired social or occupational functioning.

It is important to clearly distinguish any neuropsychiatric impairment due to alcoholism, which has been claimed as the most common cause of cerebral atrophy, from that due to HIV infection. The former is perhaps more likely.

The treatment programme of someone with alcohol dependency consists of an assessment of the drinking pattern, personal, social and physical problems. It should if possible involve a spouse or partner, with a treatment plan to decide whether complete abstinence is desirable, or whether controlled drinking is feasible.

In longer term treatment, psychological interventions are required, with behavioural methods, group therapy and education, and the use of agencies specifically designed for patients with HIV infection and alcoholism. It has been found clinically that it is extremely difficult for patients to join the general alcohol services, such as Alcoholics Anonymous, and to disclose their HIV status in these settings. Therefore, services specifically for patients with HIV and alcohol problems have been developed.

10.5 How might patients with personality disorders and HIV infection be recognized and best managed?

The diagnosis of a personality disorder is difficult and contentious, and there may be no valid diagnostic categories of personality disorders, but rather a number of unrelated disorders. However, psychiatry does presume a major category of personality disorder, defined as deeply ingrained maladaptive patterns of behaviour recognizable in adolescence or earlier, continuing throughout most of adult life, and leading either the patient or others to suffer, with an adverse effect on the individual or society. It is of prime importance to clearly determine that there is no other psychiatric diagnosis to account for the presenting behaviour of the patient, for example, an affective disorder.

Management of a patient with personality disorder and HIV infection is extremely important in terms of containing anxiety of both patient and staff involved. It requires careful boundary setting and clear communication between colleagues involved with the care of the patient, in order to provide the optimum medical care. Patients may suffer from self-detrimental impulsivity with unstable intense relationships, identity confusion, shifts of mood and chronic lack of enjoyment of life. This may be associated with self-mutilation, eating disorders and sexual promiscuity. A clearly defined regular contact with a healthcare worker can contain some of the patient's disturbance and limit potential damage caused by these behaviours. It may be necessary to obtain specialized help and supervision.

It is extremely important to continue to rule out any subsequent organic or psychiatric disorders, thus ensuring that the problem is persistent since adolescence and not episodic.

Careful management will enable patients to have a more stable lifestyle with benefits to their physical health, including regular clinic attendance, appropriate medication, and limiting risk of infection and transmission to others.

10.6 What is the significance of functional psychosis in patients with HIV infection and how is it best managed?

Mania is recognized as occurring occasionally in patients with physical illnesses, and in patients with HIV infection, and can be a result of disease progression. It is not yet clear what specific factors contribute to the occurrence of mania.

The mania may be a consequence of the illness, biological and psychosocial, and it may be coincidental to the illness, for example, a patient with a strong family history of manic illness or previous episodes. Acute infections may present as a manic psychosis before, or instead of, appearing in the more classical acute organic brain syndrome form. It is therefore wise to arrange for appropriate investigations in patients with HIV infection and psychosis, that is, for a full neurological examination and for computed tomography (CT) and magnetic resonance imaging (MRI) to exclude secondary infections. The management of patients with mania is the same as in general psychiatric practice, but with the added complication that patients with HIV infection appear to be especially sensitive to the side-effects of major tranquilizers, such as phenothiazines (e.g. chlorpromazine) or butyrophenones (e.g. haloperidol). There have been reported cases of acute dystonic episodes on low doses of haloperidol and extrapyramidal side-effects are frequently reported. It is wise to start on a low dose of haloperidol and to observe closely for side-effects whilst carefully excluding causes of the mania, e.g. drugs.

The psychodynamic contribution to a manic episode, in a patient with unresolved issues brought into crisis by the illness, is very important to assess alongside the biological factors.

10.7 What is AIDS dementia complex? How does it present and how is it best managed?

AIDS dementia complex is the progressive loss of cognitive and intellectual function which has been clearly defined in individuals with AIDS. Present prevalence appears to be between 6 and 10% of large population samples of people with AIDS. It is related to the final stage of illness, but may be the only AIDS-defining disorder in a patient with end-stage disease.

If one believes in the concepts of cortical and sub-cortical dementias, then AIDS dementia complex belongs in the latter category. In most patients, disorders in three areas of mental functioning can be defined — cognitive, motor and behavioural. The early symptoms of patients with AIDS dementia complex are non-specific. It is sometimes impossible to differentiate between an individual with a depressive or anxiety disorder and an individual who is beginning to develop this progressive dementia. Symptoms are seen in all three areas and, although the patients themselves may not recognize a change, friends may comment on alterations in behaviour and personality 4 or 5 months before presentation. Common symptoms are those of mental slowing, inability to do things as quickly as before and apathy followed by global intellectual impairment. The mean prognosis time from diagnosis of AIDS dementia to death is 9 months. The motor abnormalities which tend to accompany the AIDS dementia, such as ataxia, are indicative of global central nervous system (CNS) impairment.

It is important to exclude acute secondary infections which are potentially treatable, such as toxoplasmosis. Therefore, all patients presenting with some form of neuropsychiatric impairment, as described above, should undergo thorough investigation, including CT and MRI. AIDS dementia complex is believed to be caused directly by HIV. As the condition progresses, the differentiation from other psychiatric states or other CNS opportunistic infections becomes easier, because the doctor is assessing the same patient over a period of time. At later stages the dementia is a global dysfunction with loss of memory, attention, language and praxis. The individual will eventually lose the ability to speak and will be mute, bedbound and incontinent. In late dementia, 30% of patients will develop a myelopathy or spinal cord dysfunction. There are then signs of diffuse cognitive dysfunctions such as frontal release, for example, grasp reflex.

There is a typical pattern of radiological abnormality that is seen in up to 70% of patients with late dementia. The ventricles become enlarged with severe atrophy in a widespread pattern, more marked in the frontal temple areas, and the white matter appears attenuated and rarefied. In terms of neuropathology, the main damage appears to be to the deep white matter and sub-cortical nuclear groups, such as the thalamus and sometimes the brain stem, but the white matter is most severely affected with the cortex often being spared. Occasionally, focal areas of abnormality can be seen where there is more prominent inflammation or collections of inflammatory cells. The most important marker for AIDS dementia complex within the brain is the presence of multi-nucleated giant cells within the white matter.

10.8 What is the value of neuropsychological testing to determine early AIDS dementia complex?

There has been widespread use of neuropsychological testing or psychometric testing in order, firstly, to have a clear standardized marker for cognitive impairment and, secondly, to recognize if there are specific patterns of neuropsychological dysfunction which will be important in diagnosis. Patients' subjective opinion of their memory and concentration does not correlate well with their neuropsychological performance in real life. The closest correlation with subjective memory loss is depression and anxiety.

Psychometric testing looks at various cognitive abilities, such as attention span, short-term memory, long-term memory, speed of reaction etc. It appears that psychomotor slowing, memory, attention and concentration are the spheres of cognitive functioning which seem to be affected earliest in patients with AIDS dementia complex. An example of the test for psychomotor slowing is that of the grooved peg board. The patient is asked to put pegs into a series of holes in the board, in sequential order, as quickly as possible. They are timed on this task with dominant and non-dominant hands. Other examples of tests include trail making, such as joining up a series of numbers as quickly as possible with the pen not leaving the paper, and then joining up alternate numbers and letters, again with the pen not leaving the paper. Attention and concentration are tested in a number of psychometric tests alongside other cognitive functioning, e.g. digit span. Memory can be tested with recall of a piece of prose after 1 minute and then after 20 minutes. A standard instrument is the Wechsler Adult Intelligence Scale.

It is important to note that there are numerous reasons for variations in psychometric test results, for example, education, practise, alcohol and drug use. Perhaps their greatest value is in terms of prospective follow-up of a patient with suspected cognitive decline. Novel techniques such as the EEG which gives neurophysiological markers of AIDS dementia complex, and MRI which measures neuronal loss, may be a step forward in reducing the bias inherent in psychometric testing in detecting early dementia.

10.9 What is the risk of suicide in patients with HIV infection and how should this be assessed?

Suicide is increased up to twofold in patients with a potentially fatal illness such as cancer. Population studies have shown that patients who have committed suicide are more likely to have had a recent physical illness. It is therefore not surprising that patients with HIV infection may have a higher risk of suicide. In addition, the level of psychiatric morbidity in patients with HIV infection puts them at further risk of being a group liable to commit suicide.

It is extremely difficult to know exactly the rate of suicides in patients with HIV infection. This is a population with very high natural morbidity. An individual may have died of drug overdose, but may be presumed to have died of a severe infection. In the intravenous drug user population, deaths from intentional drug overdose can be misclassified as accidental rather than suicide. Suicide is a rare event, and therefore prospective studies would take many years with large population samples. If studies are done at autopsy, there is a doubt over seroprevalence unless this is routinely done, and also limited data on persons at risk. Many studies are therefore retrospective and on clinical material which has rich information but perhaps reduced representativeness. The questions asked are: 'is HIV a catalyst of suicidal behaviour or an inducer?', 'do persons at risk of HIV infection derive from a population already at risk of suicide on the basis of other pre-morbid risk factors, for example psychiatric history or history of deliberate self-harm?', and 'is it possible to identify risk factors most predictive of suicide morbidity?' It is suggested that there are temporal relationships, such as the onset of AIDS-related illness, or an HIV/AIDS diagnosis with suicidal behaviour. Others believe that cumulative stressors that build up over time, such as multiple bereavements and illness amongst close friends, physical debility etc., lead to suicidal behaviour.

A study of suicides amongst AIDS patients in New York in 1985, showed an increased risk of suicide of 36 times compared to a population of healthy men in the same age group. This needs careful interpretation because the group of suicides is not representative of men of that age group in New York. Of these suicides, 50% had a diagnosis of depression, 50% had seen a psychiatrist within 4 days, 33% had made previous suicide attempts and 25% of the suicides occurred on medical wards. They all occurred within 9 months of an AIDS diagnosis.

More recent studies in Italy on large populations of patients looking at deliberate self-harm and attempted suicide, show that HIV-positive individuals with psychiatric history or a history of deliberate self-harm had increased suicidal behaviour, and that it was psychiatric history and a history of attempted suicide that were the greatest predictors of present suicidal behaviour. The risk was seen to be highest either within the first 6 months or after 3 years of an HIV diagnosis. It may be that these represent two different groups of patients — those who have a heavy load of psychiatric predisposition for whom the HIV diagnosis is the final catalyst towards suicide, and those who decide to end their lives in response to worsening illness.

There is also much debate about patients' autonomy with regard to euthanasia in the situation of worsening debility from HIV infection and no effective treatment. For some patients, it may be a rational decision to choose not to have further invasive medical treatment. Others may take this one step further in wishing to actively end their lives before they become overly dependent on other people. However, for other patients it is clear that a mood disorder is present, and mental state examination is extremely important to exclude a diagnosis of clinical depression and to treat this where it applies.

The management of such patients is complex and must depend on many matters, such as their current physical and psychiatric state, and the opinions and feelings of friends and relatives. It may be necessary to discuss with psychiatric colleagues and approved social workers whether the application of the Mental Health Act appears appropriate in particular cases where a psychiatric diagnosis can be made.

10.10 Is there evidence of cognitive impairment in early HIV infection?

Ever since the discovery of a dementing process associated with late-stage AIDS, there has been some concern that this is a progressive process beginning early in HIV infection and causing functional cognitive impairment in asymptomatic HIV-positive patients. In large-scale prospective longitudinal cohort studies of patients with early HIV infection and matched controls, this has now been clearly refuted. There is no significant difference between the cognitive performance, as tested on a battery of neuropsychometric testing, of HIV-negative subjects and HIV-positive asymptomatic subjects. However, there are a small number of HIV-positive asymptomatic subjects who will exhibit some cognitive changes, and these people may show impairment in particular scales such as those measuring reaction times. There is no indication, as yet, that they will progress to dementia. Other factors complicate the picture — intravenous drug use, alcohol use, education etc. On this basis therefore, it is clear that individuals should not be discriminated against in terms of employment prospects or ability to drive etc. as a result of HIV infection, and that cognitive impairment in a functional sense is linked to end-stage illness, in a small percentage of patients, and not the asymptomatic stage.

Patients frequently complain of memory loss and concentration loss, and if they have heard reports of AIDS dementia complex they can be extremely concerned that they are showing the first signs of cognitive decline. Most studies indicate that subjective loss of memory and concentration is a sign of depression or anxiety rather than cognitive impairment, and that there is little correlation between subjective memory loss and real neuropsychiatric impairment. A mental state examination would be required, and the patient should be reassured that such memory loss is common at times of stress.

10.11 How does one classify patients who repeatedly seek HIV testing despite negative results and lack of behaviour that would put them at risk of contracting HIV infection? How are such patients managed?

These patients have been referred to as the 'worried well', although this term is misleading to the extent that often these patients are far from well in terms of their psychiatric status.

Studies have indicated that 30% of outpatients in sexually transmitted disease clinics, present primarily with hypochondriacal fears and psychogenic pain. Patients have always presented at genitourinary clinics with the morbid conviction that they have symptoms of sexually transmitted disease, e.g. syphilis or gonorrhoea. In the context of HIV, this group of patients has been called the 'worried well'. This is a group of people without HIV infection for whom the virus has become a vehicle for the expression of general psychological vulnerability and sexual guilt. These patients can be distinguished from those presenting with what we have called AIDS anxiety, this being an anxiety or awareness of the potential risk of exposure to HIV which has been heightened by media coverage, but which is effectively ameliorated with appropriate information, discussion, counselling or stress management. People known as the 'worried well' are similarly motivated, but they do not respond over the long term to discussion, counselling, stress management and reassurance that they are not at risk.

Within the term 'worried well' there is a spectrum of psychiatric diagnoses. It is therefore extremely important to make the correct diagnosis in order to instigate appropriate treatment. A study of such patients at the Middlesex Hospital Medical School found considerable consistency in their presenting features. They all suffered from an unshakeable anxiety-laden conviction that they had HIV infection, interpreting the presence of somatic anxiety symptoms such as fatigue, sweating, shaking, rashes, muscular pain, intermittent diarrhoea, sore throats, slight weight loss, etc. as signs of HIV infection. About half of them also had panic attacks triggered either by media programmes on AIDS or the anxiety symptoms themselves, or involuntary obsessional thoughts about AIDS. This is a consistent feature, the appearance of obsessive, compulsive symptoms, chronic ruminations about HIV with images or thoughts, involving punishment for high-risk behaviour, loss of loved-ones, infecting family members, etc. These could be related to serious suicidal intent. The compulsive disorders involved checking the body for lesions which could get to the point of being delusional. Depressive phenomena were present in three quarters of patients, and suicidal thoughts were present in over half of them. Background features showed sexual adjustment difficulties in adolescence, often associated with strict religious influence from family backgrounds. A high percentage of the patients had covert sexual activity only and often in the context of considerable guilt.

Management of these patients firstly requires the correct psychiatric diagnosis. This may well be the presentation of an individual with severe clinical depression or with a psychotic illness, including schizophrenia, with a delusional system which has incorporated infection with HIV. For patients presenting with a hypochondriacal state, their management presents a particular dilemma. Reassurance maintains the problem, and helps the patient to avoid tackling underlying difficulties which generate their behaviour. The treatment of choice for patients with hypochondriasis would be a behavioural psychotherapeutic programme involving strict behavioural contracting, a re-interpretation of the causes of patients' stress, response prevention to alter their behavioural response to that stress, and enhancement of their self-esteem. At the Middlesex Hospital, this has been shown to be an effective treatment for this particular patient group.

10.12 What is the usual psychological response to HIV testing and how can patients who appear to respond adversely be best managed?

Studies have been done, particularly in New York, on patients' responses to HIV testing. In samples which are about two-thirds gay or bisexual men with a mean age of 35, it was found that at recruitment for HIV testing, a quarter of the subjects qualified for a DSM IIIR diagnosis, using the structured clinical interview, mainly having mood disorders, depression and dysthymia. Other studies have found that about 30% of patients coming for HIV tests have adjustment disorders.

Anxiety and depression are comparable both for patients who are subsequently found to be HIV seropositive, and those who are subsequently found to be seronegative. In some studies it is found that seropositives show an increase in depression and anxiety upon notification, and that there is a significant difference between the positive and negative groups at the moment after notification. However, with increasing time, the reported level of depression and anxiety dropped to the same level for both, so that by 10 weeks, the two groups were comparable. However, other studies find that the seronegative group remains more anxious than the seropositive group, and this may be because they persist in being at risk of HIV infection.

The important intervention that has been present for many years is that of pre- and post-test counselling. It is essential that patients receive clear concise advice and information about HIV infection and AIDS, so that they can appreciate what it means to be seropositive for HIV and also understand the difference between this and having AIDS. Research suggests that for patients who test as HIV seropositive, there needs to be some additional counselling to enable them to adjust to their diagnosis.

Following adjustment to an HIV diagnosis, patients who are seropositive continue to have a number of events which will cause fluctuations in anxiety and depression as new psychological adjustments have to be made — to other peoples' reactions to their diagnosis, to their first physical illnesses, to being enrolled on drug trials, etc. Most studies have found a higher prevalence of psychiatric distress in intravenous drug using groups, who perhaps have more limited resources in terms of adapting to new circumstances and developing dependent relationships with medical services.

The question of suicide risk around the time of testing is important, and it should be noted that patients with previous histories of psychiatric illness or previous histories of deliberate self-harm behaviour should be carefully followed up in order to avoid missing someone who becomes actively suicidal over this period of stress.

10.13 What is the role of AZT in cognitive functioning in AIDS and ARC patients?

If an assumption is made that cognitive impairment does exist in some HIV-infected individuals in the form of dementia in late-stage AIDS, and that these individuals are without either opportunistic infections of the CNS or other systemic opportunistic infections which might affect clarity of thought, then we can presume that this cognitive impairment is due directly to the presence of HIV in the CNS. In research on the effect on cognitive impairment, it is viewed not as functional impairment or in any way like a dementia, but as very fine changes in cognitive impairment which would only be picked up with extensive batteries of neuropsychometric testing. However, some believe that those HIV-infected individuals who do finally dement may do this gradually, such that they do start with very slight impairment of their cognitive functioning. It is therefore argued that appropriate drug treatment at early stages of HIV infection may minimize or halt the dementing process.

In testing the hypothesis that progression of cognitive impairment can be prevented, careful trial designs are required. There needs to be a prospective natural history cohort with 6-monthly or yearly monitoring. There needs to be careful selection of controls, for example, the following factors need to be matched:

1. Improvement in mood through placebo effect.
2. Practise effect of repeated testing related to baseline impairment levels.
3. Non-specific stimulatory effects of the drug which would improve all performance whether initially impaired or not.
4. Improvement in physical well-being mediated by changes in the functioning of the immune system.

Controls to the placebo effect of AZT are ethically not possible given its proven clinical value. Test performance scores can be adjusted for mood effects, using statistical techniques and scales for measuring anxiety and depression. The large scale cohort studies in the USA have followed up large numbers of asymptomatic patients and have revealed only a few patients who do demonstrate changes. It is therefore going to be extremely difficult to evaluate the effects of AZT on such a small group of patients in large prospective cohorts, particularly taking into account the many confounding factors on cognitive impairment, such as mood, and drug and alcohol use, etc. However, there does appear to be sufficient evidence at present to prove that AZT protects against later stage neurological complications of HIV infection. Therefore, early treatment with AZT is preferable, and more confirmatory evidence of its protection in terms of cognitive functioning may come to light in the future.

10.14 How would one manage the dilemma of testing a psychiatric patient for HIV infection and when would this be appropriate?

Occasionally, in psychiatric and general practice there arises the dilemma of whether a patient who is unable to give informed consent should have an HIV test, because of risks to themselves and others of transmission of the infection. It is important to have a clear understanding of how knowledge of the patient's HIV status would affect assessment and treatment. Most psychiatric disorders in HIV-infected patients, especially in those who are asymptomatic, are likely to be coincidental or only indirectly associated with this viral infection. In the majority, the treatment of the psychiatric disorder is therefore unlikely to be significantly affected by knowledge of the patient's HIV status. Severe depressive disorders or paranoid states, whatever their aetiology, will receive similar symptomatic treatment. However, knowledge of a patient's HIV status may be important in the case of organic brain disorders, whether caused by the direct effects of HIV on the CNS or by problems related to immunodeficiency, such as cerebral toxoplasmosis, intracranial tumours or pneumonia. In this case, treatment of the cause as well as the symptoms of the disorder will be necessary.

The possible effects on others involved in the management of the patient need to be considered. Is there a risk of infection to the patient's sexual partner or to other patients or to staff, and would such risks be reduced if the HIV status of the patient was known? This needs to be thought through very carefully as it is not as obvious as it might at first seem. Certainly, knowledge of HIV status is not essential for giving up risky activities and may indeed not lead to this. Infection control in hospital settings is in fact more likely to be effective if the guidelines used to minimize infection are applied to all patients and not just those thought to be at risk. Indeed, the whole selection of patients thought to be at risk may lead to inappropriate assumptions about patients' HIV status. If membership of one of the transmission groups for HIV is regarded as an indicator of risk of infection, for example, being gay or bisexual, an intravenous drug user or a haemophiliac, then there are risks of putting too much emphasis on group characteristics. Only a minority of members of these groups are known to be infected. What is more important is a history of specific behaviours likely to lead to infection — unprotected anal intercourse, intravenous drug use with sharing of needles, sexual contact with individuals with HIV infection without using protective measures, etc. This would require careful history taking with sensitive handling of questions, as patients have obvious fears of revealing this information. It is particularly important for doctors to make sure that their own views about patients' lifestyles and behaviour do not interfere with their clinical judgement.

Establishing a psychiatric patient's HIV status would be desirable only if knowing it would result in clear benefits to the patient, in terms of his or her psychiatric and physical health, and lead to definite reduction in the risk of infection to others. If this is thought to be the case, then testing for HIV antibodies should be carried out with the patient's informed consent other than in exceptional cases. The patient needs to have the opportunity to consider carefully the implications of a positive test result. This advice is in line with the recommendations made by the General Medical Council 1988 and the Royal College of Psychiatrists

1989. In practise, a patient is very unlikely to refuse the doctor's suggestion of testing for HIV when this is done as part of the assessment and treatment of the patient's condition. However, if the patient refuses to be HIV tested, even after the doctor has stressed the likely benefits that would follow — adequate diagnosis and treatment of the psychiatric disorder, provision of early treatment for HIV infection and prevention of medical complications, as well as possible problems — then the patient should be reassured about confidentiality and further support should be offered. The concerns and anxiety should be explored and tackled, and the doctor will need to decide whether this is one of the exceptional cases where testing without the patient's consent can be carried out. If the doctor concludes that the patient is capable of giving consent and that testing is not imperative in order to secure the safety of individuals other than the patient, or it is not possible for the prior consent of the patient to be obtained, then his or her wishes should be respected. In a ward setting, the patient can then be managed as if they are HIV seropositive, thereby minimizing risk to staff and patients. This is especially adequate if infection control procedures are applied to all patients.

Testing without the patient's explicit consent would only be justified in very rare instances, for example, when testing is essential to avoid infection to others and where, as a result of psychiatric illness, the patient is either unwilling to give consent (e.g. a manic patient) or unable to do so (e.g. in severe depression). The reasons for testing should be clearly established. In particular, in what way the patient's treatment would be influenced by knowledge of their HIV status, what benefit to the patient could be expected, to what extent would it ensure the safety of staff or other patients, and could such safety be achieved in the absence of knowledge of the patient's test result? Such a decision to test without consent should be reached after discussion with the rest of the clinical team, preferably in consultation with a physician experienced in treating HIV infection. It should be clearly documented in the notes and, if necessary, legal advisers should be involved. It is always important to maintain suitable confidentiality about a patient's HIV status, although at the same time making it clear to the patient that certain others, such as members of community psychiatric teams, will need to know of their status if they are involved in their management.

10.15 How should healthcare staff working with HIV patients be supported?

As in all areas of medical care, it is important to care for the carers. Medical and nursing staff dealing with HIV patients show particular evidence of psychological stress and other difficulties, as has been found with other workers caring for patients with terminal illness, such as advanced cancer. In addition, dealing with a particularly stigmatized group of patients may lead healthcare staff to become omnipotent, unaware of their own limitations and boundaries, in that they expect to meet all their patients' needs and to go beyond a normal professional job. Supervision is vital to maintain such boundaries with the team.

Occasionally, workers find it helpful to meet together in a group to discuss particular patients that they are dealing with, and to use this opportunity to share their work-related feelings. This can be particularly successful if healthcare workers from different settings meet in a group outside their place of work with an independent facilitator. In this way, they can feel free to talk more openly about their relationships with working colleagues, etc. Informal support amongst colleagues in their own work setting is of use, but is limited in promoting the professional maturity of workers and their institutions.

Clear procedures on infection control methods in relation to HIV infection are important in minimizing anxieties, but they can never deal with all the irrational fears we may all face as healthcare workers dealing with an infectious illness with a fatal outcome. Whatever the intellectual knowledge on a subject, there can be emotional feelings that are embarrassing to admit, for example, worries about shaking hands, cleaning cups, etc. These fears should not be reacted to in an accusative way, as it is not always possible for staff to be rational when such basic fears are touched on. However, it can be helpful for staff to feel that they can talk about these emotions and to share the daily frustrations of their work.

The appropriate supervision and support of staff is particularly important for patients who need some consistency of care throughout their illness until their death. If carers can be helped in this way it will enable them to be committed to their work, and to be fully involved in a professional manner with patients in a way which can be maintained.

11. HIV infection in women

11.1 Do women with HIV infection have an increased chance of developing cervical neoplasia?

Yes. The association has been demonstrated between women with HIV infection who develop immunodeficiency and the development of cervical neoplasia. This includes the range of abnormalities from cervical intraepithelial neoplasia (CIN) to invasive cervical cancer. In one study of 114 women with pre-invasive and invasive disease, those women who were HIV antibody positive had more advanced cervical cancer. Amongst those with advanced disease, the median time to recurrence was only 1 month in HIV-antibody-positive women, but 9 months in HIV-negative controls. It has been further reported that 9 out of 10 seropositive women who died during the study had died from advanced cervical malignancy rather than from AIDS. This report highlights the need to manage cervical abnormalities in women with HIV infection in an assiduous manner.

11.2 Is a cervical smear adequate to detect cervical abnormalities in women with HIV infection, and if so, how often should it be performed?

There have been studies demonstrating a high false-negative rate of cervical cytology screening in women with HIV infection compared to healthy controls. This is based on the performance of colposcopic assessment in women who have had a negative smear. It is accepted outside of the context of HIV infection that colposcopy will detect a higher group of minor abnormalities than will cytological screening alone. However, these findings have led to one of two suggestions by different groups of authors. Firstly, that more frequent cytological screening, i.e. every 6–12 months, should be advised for HIV-seropositive women by Papanicolau smears. Secondly, others have suggested that annual colposcopy and cytologic screening is essential to pick up disease of the cervix. Further studies to evaluate these different regimes are in progress. Whatever the results of these studies, it has long been the case that the major problem of women who progress to invasive cancer lays in those women who have neither a smear nor a colposcopic assessment. It is important that doctors encourage all women to have cervical smears, especially those with any immunosuppressive disorder. This includes other causes of immunosuppression such as receiving steroids, having a renal transplant or malignant disease.

It is also important to recognize that, in young women who present with CIN or cervical invasive disease, that HIV infection is considered as a possible underlying cause of the immunosuppression which has contributed to the occurrence of cervical disease.

11.3 Is pelvic inflammatory disease (PID) more common in women with HIV infection?

PID is a common gynaecological condition that is associated with sexually transmitted diseases. It is important to recognize that the development of PID will place a woman at risk of developing other sexually transmitted diseases of which HIV should be considered one. In women with HIV infection who develop PID, one study has shown that they were markedly less likely to have a leucocytosis; they showed a trend towards the development of pelvic abscesses and tended to need more surgical intervention. This seems to be related to the degree of immunosuppression in an HIV-infected woman rather than to HIV infection per se.

In view of the association between HIV infection and tuberculosis (TB), it is likely that pelvic TB will occur in some women with immunosuppression. Use of endometrial sampling in HIV-seropositive women with amenorrhoea may yield this diagnosis, which should then be appropriately treated by antituberculous antimicrobial chemotherapy.

11.4 In a patient who is HIV infected, how should vaginal candidiasis be managed?

It appears that in women with HIV infection, vaginal candidiasis can be more aggressive, symptomatic and difficult to treat. It is important to examine the patient properly for signs of candidal infection elsewhere, particularly the mouth, and to search for symptoms of dysphagia associated with oesophageal candidiasis. A hierarchy of mucosal candidal infections with diminishing immunity has been described. The correct management of vaginal infection in HIV-infected women more than ever depends on making the correct diagnosis. Candida infection should be confirmed by microbiological testing. Other infections which can cause a vaginal discharge such as gonorrhoea, trichomoniasis and bacterial vaginosis should be excluded, as treatment failures are often due to the wrong treatment for the wrong diagnosis.

Once candidal infection has been confirmed, treatment should be with a topical antifungal medication in the first instance. However, in most patients with HIV infection, treatment will require systemic antifungal medication. This may be ketoconazole 200 mg twice daily for 5 days, fluconazole 150 mg orally stat, or itraconazole 200 mg stat and repeated 12 hours later. The patient should be followed up to ensure that a cure has been established and advice should be given on general measures to reduce the likelihood of further candidal infection.

11.5 Can an HIV-infected woman receive the oral contraceptive pill?

The reason that this question is asked is twofold. Firstly, there is some data to suggest that the steroids contained within oral contraceptives may in some circumstances be immunosuppressive. On the other hand, some data suggest that in certain circumstances they may also be involved in enhancing immune responses. Secondly, little data exist concerning women with HIV infection receiving the oral contraceptive pill, because the issue of contraception in HIV-infected women has concentrated on the use of barrier contraception.

Overall, current information is not sufficient to contraindicate the use of oral contraceptives in women with HIV infection if there is no other contraindication to hormonal therapy. However, patients who receive the oral contraceptive pill need to be individually counselled about the need to maintain barrier contraception with partners who are known HIV antibody negative or who are of unknown sero-status.

Another issue is the effect of oral contraceptive usage on the metabolism of other drugs and vice versa. The reduced efficacy of oral contraceptive pills has been well documented in patients receiving antibiotic therapy, particularly drugs such as tetracycline and rifampicin. Up to now however, no specific interactions between AZT and oral contraceptives have been described.

11.6 Should a women with HIV infection have an intrauterine device (IUD) inserted?

There are several reasons for caution in the use of IUDs in women with HIV infection. Firstly, there is the potential risk of rendering the woman more susceptible to ascending genital tract infections and hence PID. In women with immunosuppression this may lead to an increased chance of the development of pelvic abscesses and possibly septicaemia. Secondly, in a woman who is HIV antibody positive, the use of an IUD may render the patient more infectious because of the menorrhagia which is associated with the use of this device, as well as the possibility that the thread of the IUD may cause abrasions on the head of the penis during intercourse. The use of barrier contraception as an adjunct would be advised in such cases.

11.7 What is the effect of pregnancy on HIV infection?

Normal pregnancy causes a mild impairment of host immunity which can manifest itself with an increased virulence of certain infections. It has been suggested that this mild deterioration in immunity may hasten the speed of progression of HIV infection. However, the early studies which suggested that pregnancy may accelerate HIV infection were biased, because they were based on the identification of mothers of children who had already developed AIDS, and who were themselves at particularly high risk. Further studies have failed to show any deleterious effect of pregnancy on HIV infection. However, further follow-up of these prospective studies with larger numbers would be vital to properly and definitely answer this question.

Another way in which pregnancy might affect HIV infection is by the pregnancy-induced fall in CD4 lymphocyte count, pushing the HIV-induced loss of CD4 lymphocytes to a level below which opportunistic infections or neoplasias may become more likely. This possibility is important, because the published reports show that the development of AIDS in pregnancy is more common, especially when the index disease is *Pneumocystis carinii* pneumonia. Again, these data are biased, by the reporting of mothers who have died in pregnancy rather than those who have survived, and further follow-up studies are essential.

11.8 Does HIV infection result in spontaneous abortion?

The published data on this issue are confusing, with some studies showing an increase in the history of spontaneous abortion in seropositive women, whilst other prospective studies show no increase. It therefore appears that there is a casual rather than a causal relationship between spontaneous abortion and HIV infection.

Studies have shown a higher HIV seroprevalence in women undergoing induced abortion, rather than in those who continue pregnancy. However, women infected with HIV seem to make their decisions about termination of pregnancy or continuance on issues unrelated to their HIV infection, and there is no evidence that HIV-infected women in either New York or Edinburgh select termination of pregnancy any more often than HIV-negative controls.

11.9 Does a woman with HIV infection have an increased likelihood of developing complications in a pregnancy because of the HIV infection?

Although some studies have demonstrated an increase in conditions such as preterm labour, the need for caesarean section, antenatal infections such as syphilis, and the occurrence of low-birth-weight babies born to women with HIV infection, all were confounded by the high prevalence of illicit drug use and social deprivation in the women being studied. The lack of control groups of women with similar social deprivation and injecting drug use habits, means that HIV infection could not be concluded as being the cause of these pregnancy complications.

More recently, controlled studies, both in Scotland and in the USA, have demonstrated that if women with HIV infection are compared for pregnancy complications to groups of women with whom they are socially and behaviourally comparable, then there are scant data on which to believe that HIV per se causes pregnancy complications. However, there is evidence that there is a decrease in fetal size at birth related to the stage of maternal HIV infection. However, the birth weight itself is unrelated to whether or not the baby has been infected by HIV. Furthermore, there is no evidence that congenital abnormalities are more common in HIV-infected women. The reports of a dysmorphic syndrome associated with HIV-infected mothers have been unconfirmed by large studies, including the European Collaborative Study.

It should be noted that several studies from Africa, especially those from Zaire, Zambia, The Congo, Uganda and Kenya using control group data have demonstrated poor pregnancy outcomes in women infected with HIV, especially preterm delivery, chorioamnionitis, increased numbers of perinatal deaths and antepartum haemorrhages. A reason for the discordancy between these data and those of European and North American studies, is that the percentage of women included in the African studies with advanced HIV infection and AIDS is considerably higher. This may allow the detection of pregnancy complications associated with more advanced-stage immunosuppression and increased amounts of plasma viraemia. Furthermore, another possibility for the differences between African and other studies may be due to other problems in women with HIV infection, such as malaria, malnutrition and lack of medication availability.

11.10 What factors influence the transmission of maternal HIV infection to the baby?

HIV infection can be transmitted from mother to baby either in utero during labour and delivery or during breast-feeding. Although breast-feeding does not seem to be a major mode of the spread of HIV, data indicating when is the most likely time for HIV infection to be transmitted from a mother are scant. In vitro studies have shown that the trophoblast can be readily infected by HIV, but there is controversy as to whether this is mediated via a CD4 lymphocyte receptor. HIV antigen has been detected from trophoblast derivatives and embryonic blood cell precursors in tissues from 8-week old fetuses which have been aborted. Other studies have managed to culture HIV-1 from up to one-quarter of second trimester fetuses. In these studies, precautions have been taken to minimize the possibility of maternal cell contamination, but it is almost impossible to exclude this beyond doubt.

Although there is evidence that HIV can be transmitted early in intrauterine life, it is unclear whether this is the most common or usual timing for passage of infection. However, the early onset of features of HIV infection in some children suggest that this may occur. As further research progresses, the need to answer this question is of paramount importance if attempts are to be made to develop strategies for trying to intervene and reduce materno-fetal transmission of HIV. This might be done by the use of blocking agents such as soluble CD4, or the use of antiretrovirals such as AZT or ddI.

11.11 What is the risk of vertical transmission?

The largest study looking at rates of vertical transmission has been carried out on 419 children born in Europe. After a follow-up period of longer than 18 months, 12.9% of children were shown to have been infected. The reason for having to wait until 18 months has passed is for the definite disappearance of maternal antibodies which the infant has received passively. However, other studies have demonstrated rates between 13 and 39%. There has been a tendency for studies from developing countries to demonstrate a higher rate of transmission. Whether this is due to factors other than virological ones remains to be determined.

11.12 What factors influence vertical transmission?

There is accumulating data that HIV transmission from the mother to her infant is increasingly likely as the stage of her HIV infection advances. The clinical sequelae of this accompany the progressive immunological deterioration and an increase in p24 antigenemia and plasma viraemia. As these conditions worsen, there is an increasing likelihood of vertical transmission. A further suggestion, that it is viral load which is a determinant of vertical transmission, comes from evidence that in the first 6 months after the seroconversion illness there is also an increased tendency towards transmission. This is presumably related to a higher viral titre accompanied by less neutralizing antibody being present in the serum.

It is likely that any event during the pregnancy which increases the likelihood of a breach in the placental barrier, and/or leads to a fetal transfusion of maternal blood is likely to potentiate HIV transmission. This would include threatened abortions, antepartum haemorrhages and the use of surgical invasive procedures for fetal diagnostic tests.

11.13 Is there any test to determine whether or not an individual woman is more likely to transmit HIV infection to her fetus?

The search for specific markers to identify individuals likely to transmit HIV infection has so far not turned up any definite candidates. It has been suggested that levels of antibody to the hypervariable V3 loop of viral gp120 are predictive, but this has yet to be evaluated by prospective studies. Furthermore, cases of transmission have been documented to occur despite high maternal levels of these antibodies.

Conditions which increase the likelihood of placental damage are also associated with an increased rate of transmission, for instance, chorioamnionitis. Other studies have demonstrated a link between fetal genotype and transmission. Whether or not HLA histocompatibility antigens determine the receptor status for fetal infection remains to be seen.

11.14 What obstetric interventions might influence transmission?

It is self-evident that invasive fetal procedures which might increase the likelihood of materno-fetal bleeding should be avoided. These include cordocentesis, scalp and blood sampling, and application of scalp electrodes during labour which could all result in micro-inoculation of the fetus.

Whether or not caesarean section is protective is unclear. In theory, it may minimize the time spent by the baby exposed to cervical mucus and blood in the vagina. In the current state of knowledge, it seems that caesarean section should continue to be performed for standard obstetric reasons, and not indicated by HIV infection per se. It has been strongly suggested that antenatal treatment with AZT may be protective against vertical transmission. In the few published cases of the use of AZT during pregnancy, there is no evidence of significant toxicity or fetal damage. However, the drug is not licensed for use during pregnancy, and already there have been reports of vertical transmission occurring despite the use of the drug.

11.15 What should a woman with HIV infection be told about breast-feeding?

There is no doubt that HIV can be detected in breast milk. Furthermore, cases where the woman has been infected by an intrapartum transfusion of blood and the child then infected subsequently by breast-feeding have been documented. It seems likely that breast-feeding does carry a risk of infecting an otherwise non-infected baby. However, this risk is estimated as small, and consideration must be given to the alternative sources of food for the child if admonition to the mother to stop breast-feeding is given. In developed countries it may be that alternative sources of food are readily available, but before the advice to stop breast-feeding is disseminated widely throughout developing countries, the balance of whether or not the small number of HIV cases prevented would be offset by an increase in infant deaths from malnutrition and gastrointestinal infections must be considered.

12. Paediatric AIDS

12.1 How do children become infected with HIV?

The most obvious route of infection for children is vertically from the mother. However, early in the epidemic, up to a quarter of infected children in Africa were found to have uninfected mothers, and had presumably acquired the virus via unsterilized needles frequently used to administer antibiotics. Transmission by blood transfusion was also particularly likely in young children, perhaps because of the relatively large volume infused in relation to the baby's surface area. In the developed world the transmission of HIV via blood clotting factor concentrates was also responsible for a high proportion of children who became HIV positive.

12.2 At what stage does HIV infect the fetus?

Obviously this question is very important as the risk of HIV infection might be reduced by caesarean section, if virus transmission commonly occurred during separation of the placenta or during the passage of the baby down the birth canal.

Certainly, HIV transmission can occur much earlier than this, and cases of HIV-infected fetuses of less than 20 weeks' gestation have been recorded.

No clear studies have demonstrated that caesarean section lessens the risk of HIV transmission. However, a recent study from Africa does suggest that HIV can be transmitted at the time of birth. The second twin born to an HIV-positive mother was shown to be more commonly infected than the first.

12.3 What is the risk that a baby born to an HIV-positive mother will itself be infected with the virus?

The extent of this risk remains controversial. Perhaps the most sophisticated and long-term follow-up study is the European Cooperative Study coordinated by Professor Peckham, looking predominantly at women who have acquired their HIV through intravenous drug use. In this study, the risk of acquisition of HIV was surprisingly low at about 12%. The majority of these children had symptomatic HIV infection or were HIV antibody positive by 18 months, but there remained a small number (2.5%) whose only evidence of infection was HIV viraemia.

This is a much lower apparent rate of acquisition of HIV than studies from Africa and an American and French study, showing this to be about 30%. Many of these latter studies have been criticized for the statistical methodology employed, and either for the short length of follow-up or the relatively high default rate, and more recent studies in the western world do indicate that the rate of transmission is less than 30%.

It is possible that different rates of transmission occur in different environments with different standards of health care. Differences in transmission rate may also occur as HIV infection progresses. It is possible that women with lower CD4 lymphocyte counts, with symptomatic disease or who are antigen positive, may be more likely to transmit infection than women in the asymptomatic phase of the disease, although this has not been proved conclusively in published studies.

12.4 How is HIV detected in babies born to HIV-positive mothers?

Since IgG passively crosses the placenta, the normal enzyme-linked immunosorbent assay (ELISA) test for detecting HIV infection is frequently positive in children shortly after birth. Maternal IgG antibody levels do not wane in the child until up to 15 months after birth, and so it may take this length of time before a positive HIV test in the child can be confidently ascribed to infection. Many children of course lose their HIV-positive ELISA result much earlier than this.

IgM antibodies do not cross the placenta and, therefore, IgM-positive ELISA after birth would be indicative of infection within the child, but this test has not so far been shown to be reliably positive. Similarly, detection of HIV viraemia in the cord blood or in subsequent blood samples taken from the child would be indicative of infection, but of course most laboratories are not set up to do this routinely.

The most sensitive way of detecting HIV is the polymerase chain reaction, whereby specific sequences of HIV DNA can be enzymatically augmented many hundreds of thousands of times. Detection of HIV in one lymphocyte is therefore theoretically possible, and this has been applied to children with HIV infection. As this technology is so sensitive, particular care has to be taken to avoid false-positive results. Although the specificity of this test if very high, the sensitivity for the detection of paediatric HIV infection is not perfect in the early months of life. It is obviously crucial from a psychological point of view for the mother to be given a definitive answer as soon as possible. However, it is probably even more important to avoid giving any definitive answers which turn out to be incorrect, and therefore all tests err on the side of a very high specificity with a lower sensitivity.

IgA antibodies would not cross the placenta and must be generated within the child. This appears to be a sensitive and specific test, which can be used at the end of the first 3 months of life to give a definitive answer. However, such tests are not as yet widely available in the UK.

12.5 Is it possible to say definitively that a child is not HIV-infected without doing a test?

Virtually all HIV-positive children seem to develop symptoms within the first few years of life. Therefore it is likely that most well children over the age of 3 would not be HIV infected. However, there are reports that some children, who are apparently negative at this time in life, have developed evidence of infection at a later period between 8 and 13 years. Therefore it is not possible at present to give definitive answers to this important question.

12.6 Who must give permission for an HIV test?

Clearly the parents or legal guardians must be consulted in detail about HIV testing in children, although the doctor has a separate responsibility to safeguard the confidentiality and future interests of the child. Fortunately, these two issues are rarely, if ever, in conflict.

12.7 What are the earliest signs of HIV infection in children?

Perhaps the most common presentation of HIV infection in children is failure to thrive. Often the babies have poor growth, delay in milestones, and they may also develop a wide variety of apparently minor bacterial infections.

Despite initial reports, there is no specific embryopathy that makes an HIV-positive child recognizable at birth. The originally described abnormalities were probably associated with intravenous drug use in the mother during pregnancy, rather than the specific effect of HIV.

12.8 Why is bacterial infection so common in children who are HIV infected?

As was discussed in Chapter 3, one of the effects of HIV on the immune system is that B cells seem unable to respond to new antigenic stimuli by the normal production of antibodies. These responses are particularly important for fighting many bacterial infections. Antibodies cause opsonization which facilitates phagocytosis, complement lysis is important in a few infections, and antibody-dependent cell-mediated cytotoxicity may also have considerable importance in eradicating bacterial infection. Bacterial infection is less common in adult patients with HIV infection as they have met many of these infections before. Therefore the non-specific release of antibody which is a common early feature of HIV infection, produces adequate antibody levels to ensure that bacterial infection is not a major problem. However, in children, most of the bacterial infections are being encountered for the first time during a period in which the B cells are less responsive. Therefore infections such as otitis media, pneumonia and diarrhoea are particularly common, and although common bacteria such as haemophilus, pneumococcus and toxigenic *Escherichia coli* are responsible for such infections, the children are provenly more unwell than non-HIV-infected children with such diseases.

12.9 Why is it that children do not start to produce an antibody response to HIV until after the first year of infection?

The reasons for this long 'negative window' are not clear but may relate to immune tolerance to HIV. During fetal development, those clones of T cells which are responsive to self-antigens are specifically deleted. If HIV infection is present during the early part of fetal development, this will cause specific depletion of T- and B-responsive clones so that HIV antibodies will not develop. Antibodies and T-cell responses develop eventually, possibly associated with HIV mutations which cause sufficient alteration in antigens to make them appear different from self.

12.10 What are the common opportunistic infections in children with HIV?

The range of opportunistic infections in children with HIV are similar to adults with AIDS, but the frequency of individual infections is often very different. Many opportunistic infections of AIDS are latent, e.g. toxoplasmosis and cytomegalovirus (CMV) infection. However, children will not have had time to acquire these infections which will therefore be less common. Equally, children are exposed to certain infections very commonly during transit through the birth canal, e.g. CMV and candidal infections, and therefore neonatal thrush and primary CMV are particularly common manifestations in the paediatric age group.

Whether *Pneumocystis carinii* is a latent infection or not in adults is a subject for dispute, but the incidence of this infection as the primary manifestation of AIDS is less common in children.

12.11 When do respiratory problems occur in children?

Respiratory problems, in particular *Pneumocystis carinii* pneumonia (PCP), may occur early during the course of HIV infection prior to the diagnosis being made with certainty. This is a particular problem, as the early mortality associated with HIV infection might be reduced if PCP prophylaxis was introduced at an earlier stage.

The diagnosis of PCP is complicated by the occurrence of another common infection in childhood, also causing respiratory symptoms, known as lymphoid interstitial pneumonitis (LIP), which is very rare in adults.

12.12 What is LIP?

This is a sub-acute infection occurring in children which is almost certainly associated with Epstein–Barr infection.

12.13 How is LIP distinguished from PCP?

The presentation of LIP is usually sub-acute with the development of cor pulmonale secondary to chronic respiratory symptoms. Nodular shadowing in the parenchyma often occurs, rather than the classic 'bats wing' oedema of PCP. Patients with PCP commonly have a raised blood level of lactic dehydrogenase whereas levels are normal in patients with LIP.

LIP is often associated with marked parotid swelling which is another common feature of childhood AIDS that does occur in adults but appears to be less frequent.

12.14 How is LIP treated?

LIP responds well to corticosteroids which can often be given on alternate days.

12.15 What are the neurological manifestations in children?

The neurological changes in children are essentially similar to those seen in adults, but are perhaps more common. Immature but not mature neurones in tissue culture support the growth of HIV. 50% or more of children with AIDS have a syndrome similar to the AIDS dementia complex seen in adults. Calcification of the basal ganglia is particularly common, and a variety of spastic paraplegia and spinal cord syndrome also occurs.

12.16 What is the prognosis of HIV infection in children?

It is thought that most HIV infection in children is symptomatic, although it may be difficult to diagnose asymptomatic individuals.

Opportunistic infections appear to be particularly common within the first 2 years of life and then become less common. Early presentation with a failure to thrive and bacterial infections seems to carry a particularly poor prognosis. If the child survives the first 2 or 3 years of life, the outlook improves, and some children survive for several years. Detailed studies are at present in progress to try and provide accurate knowledge of the long-term prognosis of HIV infection in children.

12.17 What is the scale of the problem in the UK?

The present frequency of HIV-infected children in the UK is extremely low. A number of children with haemophilia were infected but these tend to be looked after in specific centres, and most of these individuals are now teenagers with presentations very similar to adult AIDS.

Most HIV-infected children in the UK at present are from ethnic minority groups, whose parents probably acquired HIV outside of this country, or are the offspring of intravenous drug users, particularly in Edinburgh. Constant vigilance is required to ensure that a major epidemic amongst children does not develop in the UK — the present figures are reassuringly low.

12.18 What treatments are available in children?

PCP prophylaxis is obviously important and may reduce the mortality in the first few years of life.

AZT is also used in children. Although its use is less well established than in adults, it has been shown to reverse some of the neurological abnormalities, and it is likely that its effects on survival are similar. Many of the early studies were done with intravenous therapy because of worries about compliance and absorption, but it appears that oral therapy is equally efficacious. The timing at which oral therapy should begin is obviously difficult, as the whole time scale of the clinical progression is markedly contracted compared with that seen in adults.

12.19 What about the value of CD4 lymphocytes in children?

One of the other major problems is establishing normal ranges for CD4 lymphocyte counts in children. It is recognized that there is a considerably lymphocytosis shortly after birth and, despite apparently very high CD4 lymphocyte counts, PCP and other opportunistic infections may occur. Tables have been constructed of 'normal' CD4 lymphocyte counts in children, and these recommendations include beginning PCP prophylaxis at a CD4 lymphocyte count of 2000 cells/ mm^3 in the first 3 months of life.

13. HIV infection and the injecting drug user

13.1 What is the prevalence of HIV infection amongst injecting drug users?

It is notoriously difficult to accurately estimate the prevalence of HIV infection amongst injecting drug users as a result of many factors, some of which are peculiar to this group of individuals, which mitigate against data collection. Such factors include the criminal status of illicit drug usage, which makes it very hard to estimate its extent, and the fact that drug users form a group of individuals marginalized by society as a whole, and hence reluctant to avail themselves of the health service.

There have, however, been many studies which have attempted to estimate HIV prevalence amongst injecting drug users which, despite the reservations posed by probable inaccuracies, have provided invaluable data. The basic message of these studies has been that rates of HIV infection amongst injecting drug users vary enormously between countries, from area to area within countries, and even from one side of a city to another.

A good example of this variation can be provided by the picture in the UK in the late 1980s, when the prevalence of HIV infection in Edinburgh was apparently in the order of 60%. Similar rates were seen in Dundee, whereas in Glasgow the rate was somewhere between 10 and 20%. London had an overall prevalence of about 13%, but this varied widely between different areas of the city, while in Liverpool only about 1% of injecting drug users appeared to be infected with HIV.

This variation can also be seen in other parts of the western world. Many prevalence studies have been conducted and show high rates of HIV infection in southern Europe, especially Italy and Spain, and in New York and Miami where rates of up to 67% have been found. Much lower rates of HIV infection were shown in northern Europe and the west coast of the USA.

13.2 What accounts for this wide variation in rates of HIV infection?

For the most part, drug users function in very small and close-knit communities. Although there is some degree of mobility between these communities, the consequences of HIV infection entering an area depend largely on the internal dynamics of the local drug-using community and external influences acting upon them.

A good example of this is the HIV epidemic amongst injecting drug users in Edinburgh. In the late 1970s and early 1980s, Europe as a whole became flooded with heroin that was relatively cheap, pure and freely available. One consequence of this was a rapid rise in the number of people injecting heroin in Edinburgh. This epidemic was noted by the authorities and the response was a general clamp down on drug users, which included police searches and arrests for injecting paraphernalia, and pressure on chemists not to sell needles and syringes to people they suspected of illicit drug usage. The result of these well-meaning initiatives was to force illicit drug users further underground and to cause a scarcity of needles and syringes for injecting drug use. Consequently, the sharing of injecting paraphernalia and the use of makeshift apparatus such as sharpened pipettes became commonplace. The result of these changes appears to be the epidemic of HIV infection amongst injecting drug users in Edinburgh in the early and mid 1980s.

In Miami and New York, the high rates of HIV infection may be explained in part by the appearance of 'shooting galleries' (places where one may rent drug injecting equipment, use it and then return it to the gallery owner for rental to the next customer) in the injecting culture of these cities.

As previously stated, drug users often live in relatively small and close-knit communities of fellow users. It is therefore important not to forget the role of sexual transmission in spreading HIV within the community. It should also be remembered that it is common for drug users, be they male or female, to sell sex as a means of supporting their habit, and this is another important factor which may affect the prevalence of HIV infection. It is therefore essential that advice on safer sex should be included in any risk-reduction counselling.

13.3 What preventative advice can I give to the drug user who does not have HIV infection?

Obviously, the best way of avoiding the transmission of HIV through injecting drug use is to avoid using illicit drugs, or at least to avoid injecting illicit drugs. This is certainly the traditional approach of the healthcare services to illicit drug use. It does, however, have to be recognized that many drug users do not wish to discontinue their drug usage, and the advent of HIV infection and AIDS has, to some extent, shifted the emphasis of drug usage from abstinence to harm minimization.

To this end, it is important to recognize that even people who express a desire to be free of drugs or to go on long-term maintenance or reduction courses of oral methadone, may relapse to injecting illicit drugs, even if only occasionally. It is therefore essential that any patient who does or has in the past injected drugs is familiar with the most effective ways of avoiding HIV infection, and it should be pointed out to them that similar precautions will protect them against hepatitis B and hepatitis C infection.

The most important piece of advice is to avoid the sharing of equipment. Needles and syringes are paramount in this category, but it is also thought that transmission of HIV through sharing the spoons used to prepare the heroin for injection is possible. The patient should be made aware of how to obtain clean needles and syringes, which may be from a local needle exchange, drugs project or a chemist who is prepared to sell them to people he suspects are using them for illicit drugs. Details from your local area will be available from the Substance Misuse Services, local HIV Coordinator or via the National AIDS Manual.

It is also important to recognize that there will be instances when the immediate desire to inject drugs will overwhelm the restraint required for waiting to obtain clean needles and syringes. In such instances, people can resort to the emergency cleaning of needles and syringes. The current guidelines are that the needle and syringe should be carefully washed with cold water to remove all traces of blood. It should then be flushed with either bleach or washing-up liquid, and then flushed repeatedly with cold water to remove all traces of the bleach and washing-up liquid. It is important to point out that clean water should be used on each occasion.

It can be useful to give general advice on safe injecting which goes beyond that of HIV prevention. It is surprising how many drug users who have been injecting for many years are ignorant as to how to inject properly. Advice should include making up the drug to be injected with sterile water, which is also available in needle exchanges and many drug projects, to inject with the smallest needle possible into the smallest vein that is easy to find.

13.4 Won't all this advice and the widespread availability of needles and syringes promote injecting drug usage and hence HIV infection?

This is an argument often levelled against the needle exchange schemes and the free availability of needles and syringes. There is unfortunately no conclusive evidence either way, but no studies in areas where needle exchanges are to be found have shown a disproportionate increase in the number of injecting drug users. The Edinburgh experience previously described has shown all too conclusively what can happen when the supply of needles and syringes is severely restricted. The fact that this is not a freak occurrence, and that dramatic epidemics of HIV infection can still occur in populations of injecting drug users, is demonstrated by the experience in Bangkok, where the prevalence of HIV infection amongst injecting drug users rose from 1% in 1987 to over 40% in early 1989. Also in New York, where political pressure has prevented the development of needle exchange schemes, there has been no noticeable effect on the numbers of new injecting drug users, and HIV seroprevalence rates are overwhelmingly high.

13.5 What advice should I give drug users with HIV infection?

First, we should consider the effects of illicit drug usage on the clinical course of the HIV infection. Many studies have been done to try to ascertain whether opiates or other illicit drugs potentiate the damage to the immune system caused by HIV infection. There is no good evidence that any drug of misuse in the pure form, with the possible exception of alcohol, accelerates the clinical course of HIV infection. Street drugs, however, almost inevitably contain high levels of impurities, some of which when injected are highly antigenic, and this can certainly lead to immune suppression. It is therefore important to make patients aware of this fact and to encourage them to consider either a maintenance or detoxification programme. The advantages of pharmaceutically pure drugs, and the desire to prevent the spread of HIV infection, have led to the increasing use of injectable prescriptions for patients with HIV infection. The drugs in common use for this purpose are injectable methadone (Physeptone^R) and diamorphine.

Patients should be informed that repeated exposure to other strains of HIV and other infective agents can have a detrimental effect on the clinical course of their disease, and therefore they should be advised against sharing needles, even with people they know to be similarly infected with HIV.

Obviously, all the advice that should be given to patients outlined in other parts of this book is applicable to the injecting drug user with HIV infection. This is especially true of counselling on safer sex issues, not only to avoid repeated exposure to HIV or other possible infective agents, but also in the case of the injecting drug user who may be working in the sex industry to finance their drug habit.

13.6 How does the clinical picture of HIV infection differ in drug users from other groups?

Fundamentally, the consequences of HIV infection are the same in people with a history of injecting drug use as in any of other so-called risk groups. There are, however, a few important differences which should be pointed out. Kaposi's sarcoma (KS) is much more common in people who have apparently acquired the condition sexually rather than by inoculation. It is seen to have a maximal incidence in homosexual men, and to be least frequent in haemophiliacs and recipients of blood products, with injecting drug users occupying the middle ground.

Bacterial infections are generally more common in injecting drug users than other people with HIV infection. This is particularly true of skin infections, bacterial pneumonias and tuberculosis (TB).

Abscesses and cellulitis are obviously commonly seen in people who inject drugs. Their incidence is again increased in the presence of the impaired immune responses caused by HIV infection. They should be treated with conventional measures.

In one study in New York, it was found that as many injecting drug users with HIV infection died from bacterial pneumonias as from AIDS-diagnosing conditions. It is important that this fact is remembered when managing an injecting drug user with HIV infection who shows signs of respiratory disease.

TB is found with increased frequency amongst injecting drug users regardless of their HIV status. The patient with HIV infection is however much more likely to develop clinical manifestations from TB than the seronegative patient.

13.7 Is there any interaction between opiates and AZT?

Just as with paracetamol, there has been much speculation that methadone will compete with AZT for hepatic metabolism, hence causing increased levels of the latter and a parallel increased risk in toxicity. Although there are few data available on the use of the two drugs together, it is now widely accepted that there are unlikely to be any serious side-effects from taking the two drugs concurrently.

There was until recently a school of thought that the potentially serious side-effects of AZT, and the poor compliance of many people with a history of injecting drug use, led to a relative contraindication for its usage in some patients. Now AZT is used in doses of 500 mg per day, which results in very few side-effects. It seems unreasonable not to make it freely available to those people with a history of drug use who wish to take it, especially as haematological monitoring can be performed when the patient returns for repeated prescriptions of the AZT.

14. Antiretroviral treatment

Refer to Chapter 2 for some of the mechanisms by which these agents work.

14.1 What antiretroviral drugs are presently licensed in the UK?

Zidovudine (AZT) is at present the only licensed therapy for HIV infection. Recently, dideoxyinosine (ddI) has been licensed in the USA for patients who are intolerant to AZT, and a license for the same indication is under consideration within the European Community.

14.2 What other drugs are near the marketplace?

Another nucleoside analogue, dideoxycytosine (ddC) is widely available but does not have significant advantages over AZT, and is less likely to be developed as a single agent against HIV. When used in combination with AZT, a marked short-term rise in CD4 lymphocytes was noticed in one study.

14.3 Is there any evidence that AZT works in HIV infection?

A clear answer to that is yes. In 1987 a placebo-controlled trial was prematurely terminated when it was discovered that patients treated with AZT, following a recent attack of *Pneumocystis carinii* pneumonia (PCP), survived significantly longer and had fewer opportunistic infections than those given placebo. In this particular study, patients with symptomatic disease (AIDS related complex, ARC) were also treated, and benefited even more than AIDS patients. In AIDS patients, there was a small rise in CD4 lymphocytes (20–30 cells/mm³ on average) which fell to baseline within 1–2 months. In the ARC patients there was a larger, more sustained rise in CD4 lymphocyte count, but within a few months this was falling as rapidly in the treated group as in the controls.

Like many other studies which are prematurely terminated, it was difficult to ascertain the long-term survival benefit of AZT. AZT does appear to improve survival by a year or more when historical controls have been compared with large numbers of treated symptomatic patients. The reduced efficiency of AZT after this period could be related to the development of viral resistance (see Ch. 2).

Although no controlled studies have been performed, the use of AZT has been extended to patients who suffer from other opportunistic infections and Kaposi's sarcoma (KS). As KS may occur at a relatively early stage of HIV infection and be compatible with survival for several years without treatment, the early use of AZT is controversial. No beneficial effect of AZT on the tumour was shown in one controlled study.

14.4 What dose of AZT should we now be prescribing?

The best dose of AZT was difficult to determine in early studies, because the minimum inhibitory concentration in vitro may not be predictive of effective in vivo drug levels. AZT is a pro-drug which is converted to the active triphosphate, and it is the intracellular levels of this compound which determine the effect of the drug. Although initial clinical studies were performed using between 1.2 and 1.5 g of drug per day, between 500 and 600 mg per day are now prescribed. The evidence for this dose reduction depends upon two studies. In one American study, all patients were given 1.2 g of AZT during the first 6 weeks and this was reduced in half the patients to 600 mg per day subsequently. The survival curves of the two treatment groups were identical, although most of the patients taking 1.2 g per day suffered from side-effects requiring intermittent dose reduction. In the second study, similar survival curves were found in Scandinavian patients treated with three different dosages of AZT. Even lower dosages of AZT (300 mg per day) have been shown to produce a fall in HIV p24 antigen in one study in the USA, but this was not conducted to confirm clinical benefit at this dose.

AZT doses in the range of 600 mg per day produce far fewer side-effects than higher doses. Indeed, in the trial of early treatment with AZT referred to later, side-effects in the group given 500 mg per day were not significantly more than those given placebo.

14.5 Does a lower dose of AZT still prevent AIDS dementia complex?

One gratifying effect of the use of AZT is that patients with early AIDS dementia complex and other neurological symptoms may improve with treatment. There has been a big fall in the apparent incidence of AIDS dementia complex in HIV-infected patients over recent years, which has coincided with the widespread use of AZT. It may be that insufficient levels of drug are present within the brain when lower doses are used systemically, because of incomplete penetration of the blood–brain barrier. However, these lower doses have been in use for more than 2 years without any apparent increase in the incidence of AIDS dementia complex.

14.6 How frequently should AZT be given during the day?

Initially it was thought important to provide smooth plasma levels of AZT by regular dosing throughout the day. It is now appreciated that the intracellular half-life of AZT is long, and that twice daily dosing regimens are probably adequate.

14.7 Should doses be modified by body weight, renal or liver disease?

Plasma levels of AZT are not widely available and even if they were, this might not give information which is relevant to drug activity. Nevertheless it probably would be sensible to use a dose of AZT based upon body weight or body surface area, but this is not done. As both liver disease and renal failure produce increased levels of AZT, dose reductions should be considered. However, modifications of dose are unlikely to be considered important until a relationship between plasma levels and efficacy and/or toxicity has been more clearly established.

14.8 What are the main side-effects of AZT?

The main gastrointestinal side-effect of AZT, nausea, can be reduced by taking the tablets with meals. Headaches are also an occasional early problem.

The most important side-effect of AZT is bone marrow suppression. Neutropenia is an occasional reason for temporary cessation of therapy, usually when the polymorphonuclear leucocyte count falls below 750/mm^3. Although AZT is an effective therapy for HIV-associated thrombocytopenia, in late disease a low platelet count can occur secondary to bone marrow suppression by AZT. Anaemia is the most common severe side-effect and can be managed by temporary cessation of therapy, dose reduction, blood transfusion or, in a small proportion of patients, by erythropoietin therapy. This drug is expensive and is only probably effective in patients who do not have a marked endogenous erythropoietin response to their anaemia.

Myopathy which occurs after prolonged AZT therapy (a year or more) is often preceded by a rise in creatinine phosphokinase (CPK). Although the frequency of AZT-related myopathy is debated as a similar condition can occur without any treatment. However the CPK levels should be monitored every 3 months after 1 year of therapy, and routine enquiries should be made about muscle pains and weakness.

14.9 What drugs have important interactions with AZT?

Glucuronidation is one of the important metabolic pathways of AZT. It therefore seemed sensible in early clinical studies to avoid drugs metabolized in a similar way, e.g. paracetamol. However, as experience with AZT has grown, it has been shown that drug interactions have been uncommon. In particular, paracetamol, when taken in small doses as a minor analgesic, does not cause any untoward interaction.

The most important interactive toxicity between AZT and other drugs appears to be because of additive bone marrow toxicity, e.g. in the treatment of cytomegalovirus (CMV) infection with ganciclovir. However, other potentially bone marrow toxic drugs, such as co-trimoxazole, appear to have little additive toxicity.

14.10 What is the role of AZT in early treatment?

This remains a complex subject and some of the studies which will hopefully clarify this issue, such as the Concorde study in the UK and France, are still under way. AZT and placebo were compared in two studies in the USA of asymptomatic patients or in patients with mild early symptoms of HIV infection. These studies were stopped prematurely as significantly reduced numbers of patients in the treated groups progressed to AIDS. There was also a tendency for AZT to prevent the downward drift of the CD4 lymphocyte counts observed in the placebo group. The premature termination of these studies has been criticized because it was not established whether the reduced frequency of AIDS would lead to improved survival in the treated group. As less than 20% of patients showed any progression in either study, if early treatment is adopted, a relatively high proportion of patients would receive a potentially toxic drug with no obvious short-term benefit. However, the toxicity in the 500 mg AZT-treated group was low.

Another study performed by the Veterans Administration was also terminated early. In this study, all patients received AZT when their CD4 lymphocyte count fell below 200 cells/mm^3 or they developed AIDS. Although the group initially treated with placebo developed AIDS more quickly than the group originally given AZT, the survival in both groups was identical. Although there was no apparent survival advantage for patients given AZT at an early stage of disease compared with those given the drug later, these results need to be interpreted with caution, as the number of non-AIDS-related deaths was high and compliance may have been poor in both groups.

Recently, preliminary data from the MRC Anglo-French Concorde Study has provided further information on the use of AZT (compared with placebo) in patients with asymptomatic HIV infection. This study reports no difference in the frequency of disease progression or mortality between those who were randomized to receive AZT at the start of the trial, compared to those who deferred taking AZT until they developed clinical symptoms. Despite the failure of this study to demonstrate a significant clinical benefit to those patients receiving earlier AZT whilst asymptomatic, there was a significant difference in the CD4 lymphocyte counts in those patients who received AZT rather than placebo. Although the results of this study appear to be at odds with those of the two American studies, this is not necessarily the case at all. The importance of the MRC continuing for a full 3 years with the Concorde Study, is that it examines the longer term follow-up of patients involved than either of the previous studies. Thus, it may be that the short-term benefit previously observed, which resulted in the premature termination of the American studies, has been shown to be only a transient phenomenon by a longer period of follow-up.

The data so far leads to the clear conclusion that clinical studies using combinations of antiretrovirals in early disease must be rigorously carried out with adequate periods of follow-up for patients enrolled. Further MRC trials, such as the Delta Trial, involving combinations of AZT with ddI or ddC are in progress. Similarly, trials combining nucleoside and non-nucleoside analogues (e.g. TIBO-L, Nevirapine) have been given an added urgency by the data that a single antiretroviral agent does not offer significant advantages to patients with early asymptomatic HIV infection.

14.11 What is early treatment?

The studies of early treatment were too small to demonstrate benefit for patients with a CD4 lymphocyte count above 500 cells/mm³. Indeed, progression to AIDS was probably prevented mainly in those with a CD4 count of less than 350 cells/mm³. Most British clinicians who favour early treatment would discuss the pros and cons of this therapy with asymptomatic patients who had a CD4 lymphocyte count of about 350 cells/mm³.

The licensed indication for the use of AZT in asymptomatic patients in the UK, includes those with a rapidly falling CD4 lymphocyte count. It is possible to identify retrospectively patients at increased risk of AIDS, because of a rapid decline in CD4 lymphocyte count. However, it is unclear whether this rapid fall of CD4 lymphocyte count can be identified prospectively.

14.12 What about AZT resistance and early AZT treatment?

One worry about early AZT therapy is that it might encourage the develop-ment of drug resistance. In fact, only intermediate resistance (the virus remaining sensitive to less than 1 μmol of drug in vitro) has been shown so far following early treatment. Resistance takes longer to develop with patients treated early in disease compared with those treated when AIDS has developed. This pattern is reassuring for those clinicians in favour of beginning AZT treatment at an earlier stage. In any case, there are no definite data to connect viral resistance with loss of clinical effectiveness.

14.13 Does AZT treatment work in patients with very advanced disease?

There is increasing evidence that even with advanced HIV infection and very low CD4 lymphocyte counts, AZT continues to provide survival benefit. Patients should therefore be encouraged to take the drug if possible, even in small doses.

14.14 Are there data to support the view that ddI is an effective antiretroviral agent?

There are no direct data showing in a placebo or a comparative control study that ddI improves survival in HIV-positive patients, although comparisons with AZT are now in progress. Phase 1 and 2 studies do show improvements in the same surrogate markers (CD4 lymphocyte count and HIV p24 antigen), which predicted the usefulness of AZT in such patients. As changes in surrogate markers may not predict increased survival, their use to determine whether antiretroviral agents are useful remains hotly debated.

14.15 What are the major side-effects of ddI?

ddI has a different side-effect profile to AZT, causing diarrhoea, pancreatitis and peripheral neuropathy.

The diarrhoea is more common in AIDS patients and in those with pre-existing symptoms. Newer ddI formulations should reduce, but not obviate, this side-effect.

When peripheral neuropathy occurs, it affects the lower limbs and is painful. It usually reverses on stopping ddI therapy, and again is more common in late disease.

Pancreatitis, which may produce a major metabolic upset and even death, is far more common in late disease. How frequently pancreatitis is due to ddI is not clear, as the frequency of pancreatitis with HIV infection per se is unclear. There appear to be no clinical predictors, such as the development of mild abdominal pain or a raised amylase, which presage the development of this serious complication.

14.16 When should ddI use be considered?

An alternative drug should be considered in those patients unable to tolerate AZT because of side-effects. In addition, many patients appear to deteriorate 1–2 years after AZT treatment has been started, and they and often their doctors are keen to try an alternative drug in the belief that the virus has become resistant to AZT. ddI is now available in the USA and is widely used in these two situations.

ddI is also available in the UK for compassionate use. As reappearance of AZT sensitivity in virus previously resistant has been shown following ddI administration, patients should perhaps be given the opportunity to continue AZT if they possibly can while they start ddI.

14.17 What about other drugs?

There are a number of other compounds which have anti-HIV effects. One of these, Foscarnet, acts directly on the reverse transcriptase and has activity against viral DNA kinases. It is used in HIV-infected patients, primarily because of its value in the management of CMV infections. Like ganciclovir, the other major anti-CMV drug, Foscarnet has to be given intravenously. One controlled study comparing these two drugs in the treatment of CMV retinitis was prematurely terminated because of a clear survival advantage for Foscarnet, perhaps because of its antiretroviral effect or synergism with AZT. This has led some clinicians to believe that Foscarnet is the treatment of choice for CMV infections. As the survival of patients with CMV infection is relatively short (6 months), quality of life must be more important than small improvements in survival. Thus it is likely that choice of treatment will continue to be governed by side-effects and patient tolerability.

As the viral protease of HIV has now been crystallized, protease inhibitors have been constructed which have no effect against the mammalian enzyme and are therefore unlikely to be toxic. At least one of these protease inhibitors is in Phase 1 clinical study.

A novel group of safe derivatives of benzodiazepine, which inhibit reverse transcriptase, was discovered by Paul Jansenn in Belgium. Interestingly, such compounds only inhibit the reverse transcriptase of HIV-1 and not HIV-2, and so are thought to act by distorting the overall shape of the enzyme. Unfortunately, resistance rapidly develops following mutations within the *pol* gene. Fortunately this resistant virus remains sensitive to AZT.

14.18 Why may combination treatment be helpful?

Combination treatment may prevent the development of viral resistance, as several mutations would have to occur simultaneously in the virus to allow it to grow in the presence of two drugs. It may also be possible to use lower doses of drugs in combination and so reduce toxicity. This latter effect appears less likely as, in limited clinical experience, the standard dose of AZT (600 mg per day) has been required to produce optimum benefit on surrogate markers.

14.19 What are the best combinations?

It would be attractive to have a combination of a drug which acts early in the viral life cycle and one that acts at a much later stage. Those drugs acting early prevent new infection of cells, as they inhibit reverse transcriptase and so inhibit the formation of the viral DNA template. Those drugs acting late prevent productive viral replication in an already infected cell. One such potential combination already exists, viz interferon, which acts by preventing budding of virus from cells, and AZT, a reverse transcriptase inhibitor. However, initial studies of this combination indicate that the dose of the two drugs is limited either by bone marrow toxicity or hepatic toxicity. Additionally, the dose of interferon required for an anti-HIV effect is associated with marked side-effects which, although not serious, greatly interfere with the quality of life.

14.20 What other combinations have so far been tried?

It might be expected that nucleoside analogues would not be helpful in combination as they all act at the level of the reverse transcriptase. In fact, in vitro they appear to be additive or synergistic in their ability to inhibit viral replication, and the loss of sensitivity to AZT is not associated with resistance to other nucleosides except AZDU (see Ch. 2.) Resistance to ddI, however, does show cross resistance with ddC. Recently it has been suggested that a concerted approach using several drugs (including AZT, ddI and a non-nucleoside analogue) may produce multiple viral mutations which render the virus incapable of further replication.

A number of nucleoside analogues have therefore been used in combination. One published study indicates a higher than expected CD4 lymphocyte count rise when AZT and ddC were combined, which was sustained for the duration of the study. Unfortunately, the comparator dose of AZT was much lower than that used in clinical practice. Large-scale studies of ddI/AZT and ddC/AZT combinations are now in progress.

14.21 What of the future?

Clinicians are anxiously awaiting the outcome of the Phase 1 studies of protease inhibitors, because these might be very effective anti-HIV agents, and also because they will be attractive to combine with drugs acting as reverse transcriptase inhibitors.

It is also hoped in the future that as well as antiretroviral combinations, a combination of effective agents with immunostimulants might improve the prognosis of HIV-positive individuals.

However, it is likely that in the foreseeable future, the improvements in prognosis will continue to be small, and will be composed of minor changes in survival from better treatment of various opportunistic infections and better use of antiretroviral therapy.

15. Other therapies used for patients with HIV infection and AIDS

15.1 I have a patient with oral candidiasis, how should I treat him?

The mode of treatment will depend on the degree of severity of the candidal infection. A solitary lesion in the mouth may well resolve easily with the use of nystatin pastilles or amphotericin lozenges to suck 3–4 times a day. This should be associated with a thorough review of the patient's oral hygiene and the addition of an antiseptic mouthwash.

If the oral lesions are more extensive or if the patient is complaining of any degree of odynophagia or dysphagia, then systemic therapy is indicated. It is accepted practice to use ketoconazole 200 mg twice daily for 5 days in patients with normal liver function and no history of hepatic disease. In those with previous hepatic problems, itraconazole 200 mg daily would be indicated. However, in patients taking rifampicin, H_2 receptor antagonists, omeprazole, antacids or phenytoin, then fluconazole 50–100 mg per day would be indicated. It is our current practice to treat for 5 days and not to offer continuous medication. Some recent reports have suggested that 200 mg of fluconazole stat is an equally efficacious form of therapy. The side-effects of these triazole medications are gastrointestinal disturbances, headache, skin rash and abnormal biochemical liver function tests, which need to be monitored if long-term therapy is indicated.

At present, maintenance therapy is only offered to patients who have recurrent candida despite episodic treatment, and who find that recurrence is interfering with the maintenance of an adequate oral food intake.

15.2 In what ways can acyclovir be a useful drug for patients with HIV infection?

Firstly, acyclovir can be prescribed as a medication against herpes infections. For immunocompromised patients, recurrent genital or orolabial herpes simplex virus infection can be debilitating. Episodic therapy during recurrences or, for those with more frequent recurrences, continuous prophylactic medication can greatly improve the quality of their lives. Episodic therapy is usually given as 200 mg 5 times daily for 5 days and prophylactic therapy is normally quite efficacious at 400 mg twice daily. At these doses, side-effects are rare, although gastrointestinal disturbances and rashes may occur.

Another herpes virus, the varicella zoster (VCZ) virus causes shingles when it reactivates. Treatment with 800 mg of acyclovir 5 times daily is efficacious in reducing the duration of and improving the healing of lesions. Whether or not severely immunosuppressed patients who have frequent recurrences of shingles would benefit from prophylactic acyclovir is uncertain at present.

Another herpes virus, cytomegalovirus (CMV) has been suggested as both a cofactor for progression of HIV-associated immunosuppression, as well as causing disease in immunocompromised patients in its own right. A study to evaluate whether or not acyclovir at 800 mg 4 times a day could reduce the frequency of CMV infection in patients with AIDS, showed no protective benefit. However, this study did suggest a possible benefit of acyclovir for patients with AIDS.

Secondly, it has been suggested by the latter study that survival of patients with AIDS is longer in those who receive acyclovir medication continuously. The mechanism of action of this survival benefit is unclear. There is no evidence that acyclovir has a direct anti-HIV effect. It has therefore been suggested that acyclovir may be acting on other viruses, including herpes simplex, CMV, Epstein–Barr and VCZ, to inhibit their putative role in the pathogenesis of the HIV-induced immunosuppressive disorder which leads to AIDS. Further evaluations in clinical trials, both in patients with earlier and later stages of HIV infection, will answer this interesting question.

15.3 Should a patient with suspected *Pneumocystis carinii* pneumonia (PCP) receive steroids?

There is evidence that patients with severe PCP infection causing a considerable degree of hypoxia (PaO_2 of less than 8 kPa) benefit from receiving intravenous methyl prednisolone 40 mg 4 times a day. The mode of action of this is believed to be in reducing the inflammatory response in the lungs, leading to less blockage of small alveoli by inflammatory exudates. During this steroid course it is advisable to add isoniazid to cover the patient against developing *Mycobacterium tuberculosis* infection in their already immunocompromised lungs. Clearly, there are important considerations in giving steroid medications to patients who already have cell-mediated immunosuppression. It is vital that the course of steroids is as short as possible and that the doses are reduced in a standard stepwise manner.

15.4 If patients are allergic to Septrin, what medications can they receive when they develop PCP?

One option is clindamycin 600 mg 4 times a day plus primaquine 30 mg per day. This course is normally given for 2–3 weeks. Primaquine's side-effects are predominantly methaemoglobinaemia or a haemolytic anaemia (especially in those patients who are glucose-6-phosphate dehydrogenase (G-6-PD) deficient), nausea and vomiting. Clindamycin can cause gastrointestinal disturbances with diarrhoea which should lead to the search for clostridium toxins. Hepatotoxicity should lead to the monitoring of liver function tests in patients receiving long-term therapy.

Alternatively, pentamidine may be used as PCP treatment. In very mild cases, a 14-day course of 600 mg pentamidine isethionate inhaled once daily should be an acceptable form of treatment. For moderate to severe PCP, 4 mg/kg intravenous pentamidine isethionate is added once daily to the inhaled medication for the first 3 days of therapy. Additional doses of intravenous therapy are given on alternate days following the 3 day initial induction course. The adverse effects of intravenous pentamidine are nephrotoxicity, postural hypotension, hypo or hyperglycaemia, hypo-calcaemia, leucopenia, nausea and vomiting, and abnormalities in liver function tests. Inhaled pentamidine can cause severe bronchospasms, and pre-dosing with a bronchodilator such as salbutamol is indicated. Many patients find inhaled pentamidine produces an unpleasant taste which lasts for some time and may cause anorexia.

During intravenous therapy, it is vital to monitor blood glucose, renal function, urea, electrolytes and liver function tests. When giving inhaled pentamidine for the treatment of PCP, it is useful to monitor peak flow to check on the bronchoconstricting effects of daily inhaled pentamidine therapy.

15.5 A patient of mine has been diagnosed as having CMV retinitis and has been discharged home on maintenance therapy. What is this?

The data suggest that following an episode of CMV retinitis, patients will, if untreated, suffer a recurrence in about 50 days. Recurrences of CMV can lead to ever increasing loss of vision with eventual blindness. It is therefore important to try to prevent any further degree of visual loss by the use of maintenance therapy. The majority of patients do opt for maintenance therapy, although a minority will opt for regular surveillance of their visual fields and a fundoscopy to try to detect any early recurrences of their retinitis.

Your patient will have maintenance therapy via a Hickman, a Portacath, or another method of central venous access. This is so that one of the two drugs used in the treatment of CMV retinitis can be regularly administered. The two drugs used for this are ganciclovir and Foscarnet. Although studies using oral preparations of these drugs are in progress, no orally active, efficacious anti-CMV therapy is yet available.

Ganciclovir is given as 5 mg/kg per day in a single dose 5 days per week for maintenance to prevent reactivation of CMV retinitis. The common adverse effects of ganciclovir are leucopenia, thrombocytopenia, thrombophlebitis, fever, rash and abnormal liver function tests. Of these side-effects, the most problematic is leucopenia, especially the neutropenia which it can induce. This neutropenia is usually reversible on stopping ganciclovir therapy.

Foscarnet is given as a maintenance dose of 130 mg/kg per day with a single infusion over 2 hours on 5 days each week. An adverse effect of Foscarnet therapy is nephrotoxicity, which has led to the practice of ensuring that the patient is well hydrated during Foscarnet therapy. Any other possibly nephrotoxic drugs are contraindicated during Foscarnet therapy. Furthermore, abnormalities of calcium plasma levels have been reported. Although these are usually mild, severely life-threatening hypocalcaemia has been observed, especially when Foscarnet has been given concurrently with pentamidine. This drug combination must be avoided. Anaemia, headache, nausea and thrombophlebitis have all been reported with Foscarnet therapy. An interesting side-effect has been the development of penile ulceration in men receiving Foscarnet therapy. The overwhelming majority of the men who have suffered penile ulceration have not been circumcised. It has been suggested that the ulceration is due to a contact dermatitis, resulting from the urinary concentration of Foscarnet during excretion. During urination, Foscarnet finds its way into the sub-preputial space and a contact dermatitis occurs with resulting penile ulceration. Penile ulceration with Foscarnet cream was noted during an earlier trial when Foscarnet was being used as treatment for genital herpes simplex virus infection.

Overall, the choice between Foscarnet and ganciclovir therapies has previously been based on individual preferences as well as any contraindications, either pre-existing neutropenia or renal failure in patients with CMV retinitis. However, a recent study showed a significant survival benefit for patients given Foscarnet rather than ganciclovir. The data suggest that Foscarnet should be first-line therapy for CMV retinitis. The possible mode of action of this is the antiretroviral effect of Foscarnet, which was initially evaluated but without apparent benefit some time ago. The findings of this study have led to renewed interest in the antiretroviral effects of Foscarnet.

15.6 A patient with AIDS is taking Fansidar, one tablet daily to prevent a relapse of cerebral toxoplasmosis. Does he need to also receive PCP prophylaxis?

Fansidar consists of sulphadoxin 500 mg with pyrimethamine 25 mg. Extended use is usually accompanied by folinic acid supplementation to obviate the myelosuppressive effects of long-term therapy. The use of Fansidar as prophylaxis against PCP utilized two tablets weekly and was shown to be effective. Unfortunately, the occurrence of hypersensitivity reactions, resulting in sometimes fatal Stevens–Johnson syndrome, led to a loss in popularity for this prophylactic therapy. Owing to the long half-life of Fansidar, the allergic manifestations were enhanced and prolonged leading to a greater degree of severity than with shorter lasting sulpha-drugs.

However, in this case where the patient is tolerating Fansidar without any evidence of systemic hypersensitivity, then this will prove an effective assured prophylactic against PCP.

15.7 A patient who has had an episode of PCP has been put on dapsone prophylaxis against recurrence. The hospital notes said the blood test had been taken prior to commencing this therapy. What is the test for?

This is likely to be a test for G-6-PD. Those patients who are G-6-PD deficient are more likely to develop a haemolytic anaemia following dapsone therapy. Dapsone may be given to patients with G-6-PD deficiency, but it should be in a markedly reduced dose with constant monitoring of haemoglobin.

It is interesting that the exact mechanism of action of dapsone is uncertain, but it is thought to interfere with folic acid production. This is a similar mode of action to that of the sulphonamides to which dapsone is chemically related.

The other side-effects of dapsone are gastrointestinal (nausea, vomiting and abdominal pains) and haematological (methaemoglobinaemia, which is usually most severe in patients with G-6-PD deficiency but can occur in all patients). Other haematological problems include leucopenia and agranulocytosis. Neurological effects have been reported including peripheral neuropathy, insomnia and headaches. In patients on prolonged therapy, hepatic dysfunction has been described which necessitates the need for monitoring of liver function tests in patients on long courses of therapy.

15.8 To what extent do AIDS patients use alternative therapies?

A study at St Stephen's Clinic showed that over one-third of patients used alternative therapies at the same time as receiving prescribed medicines. These included a wide range of different approaches, from homeopathic to chiropractic, from hypnosis to aromatherapy, and a significant number of patients were buying 'alternative' therapies on the Black Market. At the time of the study, this included substances such as 'Delta T', dextransulphate and ozone therapy.

The same survey asked patients whether they felt they had benefited or not from these therapies. The overwhelming majority of patients felt they had benefited from whichever therapies they had chosen to use. Only a minority felt that these therapies had done any harm, but it was interesting to note that patients who believed in a particular therapy's efficacy usually indulged in several others to try to complement it.

Our approach is to encourage cooperation between physicians and alternative therapists. Anecdotal evidence of patients benefiting from alternative therapies is common. Many patients find that aromatherapy, massage, hypnosis, reflexology and acupuncture are very beneficial in reducing stress, focusing their energies on maintaining health and supplementing therapies which they receive from the clinic. It is vital that the patients receive correct advice, but that no-one seeks to promote or to criticize therapies without good evidence. It is unfortunate that trials have not been performed of many of the alternative therapies which patients say are so useful. However, increasingly there is a move towards evaluating the effects on immunity, quality of life and survival of alternative as well as medical therapies. It is likely that our patients will most benefit from a combined approach based on communication, improving data and reason.

15.9 If a patient chooses to stop particular medications which they are receiving, what are the usual consequences?

It depends on the class of drug which the patient is receiving and the degree of immunosuppression. Clearly, if a patient with severe CMV retinitis stops maintenance therapy, then there is a predictable recurrence of further retinitis within 3–4 weeks. On the other hand, patients with proven *Mycobacterium avium* complex infection can go months and even years with no apparent further symptoms from this infection without any therapy. A typical picture which often presents in a patient is someone who has had AIDS for 2 years or more who is receiving antiretroviral medications such as AZT or ddI, anti-PCP prophylaxis with Septrin, fluconazole for persistent and recurrent oral and oesophageal candidiasis, acyclovir because of severely recurrent genital herpes, intravenous Foscarnet or ganciclovir for CMV retinitis or colitis, and whose main complaint on a particular day is of anorexia, malaise and fatigue. It is clear that such a degree of polypharmacy is liable to lead to abnormal taste sensations, nausea and vomiting, myelosuppression with anaemia and neutropenia and disturbances in hepatic functions. Very often patients make a definite choice and choose to cease all medication. Very often, in the few weeks following this choice, they feel better, their appetite improves, and they are less dependent on the constant clock watching for when to take their next dose of tablets. In this context, psychological benefits must be considered as important as the physiological benefits. However, it must be remembered that suppressive therapies following opportunistic infections are necessary, because the immunological deficit which led to those opportunistic infections has not been reversed. The CD4 lymphocyte count and other immunological abnormalities which occur in AIDS patients are not reversed completely, either by antiretrovirals or treatment of particular infections. Therefore, it is necessary to maintain patients on continual medication to prevent the recurrence of disabling or life-threatening symptoms. It is vital that patients are appraised of the need to receive these medications, as well as making their own autonomous choice about whether they wish to continue with therapy or be supported by less toxic palliative measures. In the context of AIDS patients, it is just as vital to have this discussion with an informed patient as it is with patients with other life-threatening conditions.

16. Palliative care

16.1 When should active treatment cease in the patient with AIDS?

This is the most difficult question to answer when considering palliative care for patients with HIV infection, and leads to the most difficult dilemmas faced by healthcare professionals and those affected by the disease. For most people with AIDS, the clinical course is that of a series of potentially treatable opportunistic infections, superimposed on a background of gradually deteriorating health, often in association with parallel deterioration in social and psychological well-being. Thus, unlike the patient with an incurable malignancy, it is impossible to identify a point in the illness when symptomatic treatments become the only realistic therapeutic option. Even in the patient with one of the incurable and life-threatening malignancies associated with HIV infection, such as lymphoma or extensive visceral Kaposi's sarcoma (KS), the dilemma is seldom resolved as coexistent opportunistic infections generally develop.

In practice, the best way of addressing the problem of when to stop active treatment is to involve the patient in full and frank discussions about the progression of their illness and prognosis, encouraging them to make informed decisions about their future management.

It is useful to have such discussions electively, in an attempt to pre-empt the problems of making management decisions for debilitated patients who become confused in association with an acute illness episode, such as the patient with cerebral toxoplasmosis or the patient with marked hypoxia associated with an episode of *Pneumocystis carinii* pneumonia (PCP). If this scenario does occur, it can be useful to involve community carers who have knowledge of the patient's ability to function at home, along with their partner, family and friends, in the decision-making process.

It is important that carers working with HIV, as in other fields of medicine, accept that what is considered a reasonable quality of life is subjective and different for each individual. Thus one patient may consider generalized weakness in association with marked weight loss to be unacceptably disabling and choose to have no further acute opportunistic infections treated, whereas another patient who is blind from cytomegalovirus (CMV) retinitis and wheelchair-bound from neurological disease may still feel that they have a good quality of life and wish to have an episode of PCP actively treated. As long as these decisions are made from an informed position and in sound mind, it should be the responsibility of the attending clinicians to respect them.

16.2 Should all active treatments be stopped in the terminally ill HIV patient?

Again it is impossible to make a general rule to answer this question. Some patients may choose to stop all but symptomatic treatments and allow nature to take its course as quickly as possible; while at the other extreme, some patients may choose to continue with prophylactic therapies and even antiretroviral drugs to avoid relinquishing all hope, whilst still making the decision not to have any active management of opportunistic infections which may develop. It is also possible that a patient would decide to have some infections treated, such as an episode of CMV retinitis whilst declining treatment for another infection, such as an episode of PCP.

It can also be difficult to differentiate absolutely between symptomatic and active treatments in the context of HIV infection. For example, the treatment of oral or oesophageal candidiasis with a systemic antifungal agent, whilst being active management of an opportunistic infection, may also be considered a reasonable measure to produce marked symptomatic relief in an affected individual.

Most patients decide to occupy middle ground, and it is not unusual to see a patient who has had an episode of CMV retinitis decide to cease all active therapies excluding their intravenous anti-CMV therapy, in an attempt to preserve their remaining vision up until the time of their death. The best approach is to discuss fully the pros and cons of each therapeutic agent with the patient, to allow them to make an informed decision as to what to stop and what to continue.

This apparently rather inconsistent and haphazard approach to palliative care has been seen as unacceptable by some generic palliative care specialists, as it is at odds with the ethos of many hospices where all active management is discouraged. It is, however, the feeling of most people working in the HIV field that this approach is consistent with maximizing patient autonomy for those affected.

16.3 How does symptom control differ in patients with HIV infection as compared to other terminally ill patients?

Generally speaking, the approach to symptom control in the AIDS patient is no different than for any other dying patient. As in all cases, it is essential to take a precise history of any symptom to facilitate effective management.

As would be expected, opiate analgesics form the cornerstone of pain management. It is important to stress that other methods of pain control should not be overlooked, such as non-steroidal anti-inflammatories for musculosketal pain, radiotherapy for pressure symptoms from metastatic disease, and quinine sulphate or benzodiazepines for painful muscular cramps, all of which are commonly seen. Tricyclic antidepressants can also be useful in pain management, especially where there are associated depressive symptoms. Carbamazepine can be useful for neurological symptoms.

It should be remembered that good nursing care with the use of special mattresses, sheepskin rugs and regular turning can greatly reduce discomfort for very emaciated patients. Also, in patients with swallowing difficulties, nausea and vomiting or rapidly increased gastrointestinal transit time, subcutaneous opiates via a syringe driver are invaluable.

More unusual interventions which have proved useful for pain control include nerve blocks, acupuncture and transcutaneous nerve stimulation.

Gastrointestinal symptoms that are commonly faced include diarrhoea, constipation, nausea and vomiting, anorexia, oral cavity problems and perianal problems.

Diarrhoea is more commonly seen in people dying of AIDS than of other conditions because of the effects of gastrointestinal opportunistic infections. It can be profuse, producing volumes of up to 8 litres per day, and constitute markedly debilitating problems. Management is along conventional lines, and many of the more powerful opiates, such as slow-release morphine tablets, have been used in relatively high doses to good effect.

Constipation, nausea and vomiting should be managed as in the non-HIV patient. The use of antiemetics in combination with opiates in syringe drivers can be invaluable.

Many different interventions have been tried to combat the anorexia and weight loss seen in AIDS patients, including the use of synthetic progestogens and testosterones, but success has been poor, and the best approach is probably to use high calorie supplements in conjunction with expert advice from dieticians.

The mouth is often affected by opportunistic infections such as oral candidiasis, chronic gingivitis and aphthous ulceration. Mouth care is an essential part of nursing for the dying AIDS patient.

Perianal pain is a common problem caused either by profuse diarrhoea or recurrent intractable herpes simplex infection and this should be borne in mind.

Sweats and pyrexias are commonly seen, either as a result of the HIV infection itself or an unresolved opportunistic infection. As well as paracetamol or aspirin, corticosteroids can be useful in combating these (see Qu. 16.4).

Shortness of breath is also commonly seen in the terminal phases as a result of recurrent episodes of PCP, other pulmonary opportunistic infections or pulmonary KS. Access to oxygen either at home or in a hospice can be of great value, and nebulized bronchodilators can also produce symptomatic relief.

16.4 Are corticosteroids contraindicated in patients dying of AIDS?

Traditionally, corticosteroids have probably been under-used in the management of AIDS patients, because of concerns about their immunosuppressive effects super-added on an already markedly damaged immune system. More recently, they have been used to good effect in patients dying of AIDS. Possible benefits include increased appetite, a decrease in night sweats and general temperatures from either HIV or opportunistic infections, a decrease in oedema and hence pain associated with both lymphomas and disseminated KS, and an enhanced sense of well-being.

16.5 What about the use of analgesics in patients with a history of drug usage?

The use of opiate analgesics in patients with a history of drug usage can be a cause of concern for both the physician and the patient. Doctors may justifiably be reticent about prescribing opiates as analgesics to patients who continue to misuse them as part of a dependence. Conversely, a patient who has faced the battle of overcoming an opiate dependence in the past, may feel very apprehensive about taking such medicines for analgesic purposes.

While it is important not to dismiss other forms of pain relief, such as the non-steroidal anti-inflammatories that have been discussed in Question 16.3, it must be recognized that, in the majority of cases, there will be no realistic alternative to the use of opiates to control severe pain in the dying AIDS patient.

It should be remembered that patients with a history of opiate usage will have often developed a very high tolerance to these drugs, and it is legitimate to prescribe as large a dose as necessary to control symptoms in the AIDS patient nearing the end of their life. Research has shown that even patients who have not used opiates for many years, but have used them heavily in the past, will develop a high tolerance in a matter of about 48 hours.

16.6 Is there anything else that should be borne in mind when managing a patient dying from AIDS?

Unfortunately, society as a whole still attaches a lot of stigma to AIDS. Frequently, patients dying of AIDS will feel they would rather spare members of their family or some of their friends from knowing what they are suffering from. It is the duty of attendant healthcare workers to respect this wish, and it is always useful to clarify with the patient exactly who is aware of their diagnosis. Outside these people, it is essential to maintain utmost confidentiality.

As many people who die of AIDS are young or for other reasons unmarried, it is important to encourage the patient to make a will that fulfils his or her wishes, as in British law the next-of-kin is considered to be the nearest blood relative in the absence of a spouse. Some of the voluntary organizations listed in Chapter 18 can arrange for a lawyer to visit a patient at short notice to make a will at home, in hospital or in a hospice.

16.7 Who might be available to give support to a patient dying of AIDS at home?

Apart from the usual generic community services, including general practitioner and district nurses, there are several other options which can be considered. A patient who has one of the malignancies associated with AIDS, such as KS or lymphoma, is eligible for support from the Macmillan nurses. Occupational therapists can be invaluable in maximizing the quality of life in the end stages by the provision of various aids. In some areas where the disease is high in prevalence, there are specialist nurses, occupational therapists, social workers and home carers who can provide extra support for the patient in their home. Some of the voluntary organizations listed in Chapter 18 will also provide home support for people with AIDS.

The availability of these resources varies from area to area, and the best way of ascertaining what resources are available is to refer either to the area HIV coordinator or by consulting the National AIDS Manual.

16.8 What is available in the way of hospice care for AIDS patients?

Many of the generic hospices throughout the country receive central funding for the care of a limited number of patients dying from AIDS. As previously stated, there has been a reluctance amongst generic palliative care workers to be involved in the care of AIDS patients, partly because of the demands of facing a new challenge, and partly because of the possibility of contradictions in care with the ethos of many hospices. However, generic hospices are increasingly, and with much success, rising to the challenge. Your local hospice will be able to inform you of the policy in your area.

The London Lighthouse, Mildmay Mission Hospital, the Griffin Project Continuing Care Unit in London and the Milestone in Edinburgh all provide specialist palliative care for people with AIDS and operate national catchment areas. Also, a specialist AIDS hospice opened in Brighton at the end of 1992. Details of all these resources are given in Chapter 18.

16.9 What are living wills?

Living wills are a concept that originated in the USA, whereby a patient draws up his or her requests of how they should be managed if they reach a stage where they are unable to give informed consent. They are generally drawn up under the supervision of a solicitor and given to their attending doctor to be put in the patient notes. With the fears surrounding the possibility of developing a dementia, they have become quite popular amongst patients with HIV infection in this country.

Living wills are not considered to be legally binding in Britain. However, if requested by a patient, they can provide a useful guide to management if the need arises.

16.10 Are there any special rules surrounding the removal of the body of a patient who has died of AIDS?

No. The exact procedure is up to the individual undertaker concerned. Some undertakers are very understanding about dealing with the bodies of people who have died of AIDS. It is worth exploring the practice of local undertakers to discover the most sympathetic, as this can reduce any unnecessary stress for partners, families and friends.

16.11 How should a death certificate be completed for somebody who has died of AIDS?

If the letter of the law is to be followed, AIDS should be given as the cause of death on the death certificate. However, as completed death certificates become public property, this can cause a great deal of distress to the patient dying of AIDS and to their survivors.

Most people working in the field would consider it to be acceptable practice to write down another cause of death, such as bronchopneumonia, and to tick the box on the back of the form indicating that further information is available. If this is done, the registrar may contact the doctor who completed the death certificate, and the cause of the death may be registered in a confidential manner. Although this practice is not strictly correct, it is considered to be acceptable by all parties.

Anyone who receives an AIDS diagnosis should be reported using a code that maintains anonymity to the Centre for Disease Surveillance and Control. AIDS deaths should be similarly reported, and the Centre will forward the information to the Office of Population Census and Surveys, thus promoting complete statistics.

17. Ethical issues

The following case histories have been developed from discussions during interactive sessions at one of the regular HIV/AIDS Education courses which are run at the Westminster Hospital. Some of these cases have also been presented as short papers in Maternal and Child Health. We would like to thank Barker Publications for permitting their reproduction in this chapter.

These case histories are compendiums of both fictional and factual events which the authors have either been directly involved with or have heard about via those directly involved. We believe they illustrate many points which are relevant to the practice of medicine in general, but that HIV often serves to highlight the ethical dilemmas faced by those in clinical practice. We acknowledge that the suggested answers are merely that, and that the reader may well have better or more ingenious ways out of some of the problems. We are always grateful to hear of these for our mutual learning experience.

Case 1

You are a partner in a busy general practice situated in a large county town. After morning surgery, one of your partners comes into your surgery and closes the door. He says that he has something to tell you in complete confidence which he has told no-one else. You promise to honour this confidence. He then explains that he has tested himself via the local laboratory and found that he is seropositive for HIV infection. After informing you that he is asymptomatic, he asks your advice about whether he should continue to practise. He currently runs a family planning clinic, offers antenatal care and does a minor operations list.

17.1.1 What advice would you give him, and if you suggest that he continues to practise, would you advise that he stops any of his clinics or ceases performing any specific procedures?

Your answers will depend on whether your advice is based on the evidence that no doctor has yet been known to have infected any of their patients with HIV, or your concerns that you cannot dismiss the theoretical risk that this might happen in the future. In fact, there has been one possible report of a dentist with AIDS infecting one of his female patients in the USA, however this report (in the Morbidity and Mortality Weekly Review) remains unsubstantiated. A compromise view might suggest that he stop performing minor surgery or other procedures in which he risks injuring himself on sharps. But what about inserting intrauterine contraceptive devices (he might injure himself whilst cutting the thread), performing vaginal examinations in the antenatal clinic, or taking blood?

17.1.2 You ask him how he contracted HIV infection and he refuses to answer. What do you feel are the implications of this, and would any particular answer to this have caused you to review your answer to question 17.1.1?

Ask yourself what risk category you had assumed him to be in as you read the history: a gay man, a drug user, a haemophiliac, or a recently married young man who contracted the virus heterosexually from a previous girlfriend? Clearly, if he were a current injecting drug user this would call into question his fitness to practise, but none of the others should necessarily alter your answer to question 17.1.1.

17.1.3 He thanks you for your advice and says that he values your trust and confidence. You agree to meet again the following week to discuss all of this in more depth. After he has left, you wonder if you said the correct things and whether you could ask anyone for advice. Furthermore, you are unsure if you ought to inform any official body, like the local health authority, or the General Medical Council (GMC). What do you do?

The GMC advise that a doctor who knows himself to be infected by HIV should 'seek specialist advice'. This calls into question your acceptance that you would be his adviser, unless you believe you have enough knowledge and expertise to fulfil this role. However, who has these credentials? The answer is currently no-one, as there is no evidence, only anecdote and an absence of hard data on which to base any advice. Despite this, if you give him advice about his fitness to practise and he chooses to ignore it, then the GMC have recommended that you would then have a duty to report this to an appropriate body.

17.1.4 By the end of the day you return home exhausted, feeling pensive about all these issues. You are having dinner with your spouse (who is a dentist), who remarks that tomorrow she is going to be doing some really difficult work on one of your partners. You finish your brandy and casually ask which one. If the answer is the partner who told you he was infected by HIV, will you break his confidence and tell your spouse?

There is obviously no correct answer to this problem. At the course we run on the subject of 'HIV and AIDS', the replies from the participants have included direct approaches such as 'tell your spouse the complete story', roundabout methods including 'ask your spouse about their infection control policy and suggest that they take extra precautions (gloves, facemasks, etc.) with all their patients tomorrow', to the realistic view that 'it depends how you feel about your spouse!' Whatever your reply, the reality is that your spouse (and all other dentists, surgeons and health workers) should be using precautions designed to reduce the risk of acquiring infections (of any type) from all their patients whether they know their HIV antibody status or not.

Case 2

You are a single handed GP with a trainee, Dr X, who has been with you for 6 months. During one Friday evening surgery, Dr X asks your advice about a patient. Mr A is a 41-year-old computer programmer. He registered with your practice 1 year ago and has not attended since. That evening he had consulted Dr X complaining of tiredness, fevers, weight loss and moderate diarrhoea. On examination, Dr X had found that Mr A had lost 11 kg from the weight recorded when he was examined as a new patient. He also noted oral thrush and moderate hepatomegaly in a generally unwell-looking man. On further questioning, Mr A had revealed that he had known that he was HIV antibody positive for 3 years, but was not under any care concerning this.

Dr X tells you that he advised Mr A that he would refer him for an urgent assessment by the local physicians who were experienced in the care of patients with HIV infection. However, Mr A had insisted that he wanted to be seen at the specialist unit in the city hospital (15 miles away), who had looked after one of his friends, and that he would self-refer himself there as soon as possible. Dr X had reluctantly agreed to this and had prescribed him nystatin pastilles, written a sick certificate for 1 week and asked him to return in 5 days. The patient had also requested that Dr X did not record the details of his HIV infection in the notes as he was worried about confidentiality. Dr X had told him he must discuss this with you first.

17.2.1 What is your advice to Dr X?

You advise Dr X that a GP can legally write and keep his notes wherever he wants. Obviously it is up to each individual to decide what they would actually do in this situation. You suggest that one way to proceed is to weigh up the advantages and disadvantages. The disadvantages of not recording accurate notes might include the lack of continuity of care if the patient changed doctors, and marginalization of other members of the practice staff, such as the nurse and receptionist. Advantages could include the benefit to your relationship with Mr A by making him feel more secure, which might lead to his agreeing to you keeping formal notes in the future.

17.2.2 24 hours later, you are on call and receive a request from Ms B, another of your patients. She says she has visited her friend Mr A, and is shocked to find him so unwell. She asks if you will come and see him. What would you say to Ms B?

Although you may reasonably feel irked that Mr A had chosen to ignore the offer of an urgent local referral to go to a specialist unit, you do not know the outcome of this and to ask Ms B about this over the phone may result in a break in your confidentiality to Mr A.

17.2.3 Supposing you do decide to visit Mr A, you find him severely dehydrated and clinically septicemic. You learn that he had felt too unwell to travel to the specialist unit. You arrange immediate admission to the local hospital. The following day, you are phoned by the medical registrar who tells you that Mr A had died during the night. The following week, Ms B comes to the surgery. She is upset and angry. She asks that you tell her what Mr A died from. What do you say to her?

After a patient's death, the rights of confidentiality pass to their next-of-kin. You can honestly tell Ms B that you do not know the cause of death as full details of the hospital tests are not yet available.

17.2.4 Ms B then asks you to look at a purplish lump on her arm. She also reveals that she and Mr A had a sexual relationship about 8 years ago. What do you do now?

This clearly complicates matters. Ms B may well suspect the cause of Mr A's illness. It is probably possible to adequately investigate the possible (though rare) differential diagnosis of Kaposi's sarcoma (KS) on Ms B's arm without breaking your confidentiality to Mr A.

17.2.5 Two weeks later, you receive a letter from the Family Health Services Authority (FHSA) informing you that Ms B has made a formal complaint against Dr X for his negligent handling of the illness of Mr A. The letter of complaint states that 'Dr X did not take Mr A's illness seriously, he only gave him a sick note and some sweets to suck. When I saw Mr A the following day it was obvious to anyone that he was very sick and needed proper treatment. If Dr X had acted properly, Mr A might be alive now.' Who is responsible to answer this complaint?

In the context of an FHSA complaint, a GP trainee is seen as an employee of his trainer and consequently you will be responsible for answering the complaint. However, if the case was through the GMC or civil courts, then the trainee would be responsible for his own actions.

17.2.6 Dr X reveals that he has kept separate notes of his original consultation with Mr A. Are these personal notes submissible as evidence?

Any notes are submissible as evidence. In an FHSA case a GP may submit as much (or as little) information as he sees fit to support his case.

17.2.7 Do you feel it is justifiable to use confidential information to answer this complaint?

It would legally be acceptable to reveal any information to the FHSA. However, the moral issues would have to be considered by the individual GP concerned.

Case 3

You are a busy GP in a large city. One of your patients is a 30-year-old woman with recently diagnosed HIV infection who is hospitalized following a grand-mal fit. As a result of extensive investigations she is given an AIDS diagnosis on account of HIV encephalopathy, and is discharged home 2 months later with a full range of community support services. You and the hospital consultants continue to share her care.

After discharge from hospital, it soon becomes clear that she is driving her car (and motorbike), to attend hospital and also to help retain her independence. She had been a driver all her working life. Physically she is ambulant, and generally looks after herself. She has no immediate family. Overall, she has a degree of memory impairment and occasionally exhibits inappropriate behaviour. She continues to deny some aspects of her illness.

Despite counselling from several doctors, including a psychiatric assessment, she continues to drive.

17.3.1 What should be done, if anything?

a. Do nothing. Presumably if she has been told she should not drive and goes against this, then she is responsible for her actions. It may be important at this stage to investigate the possibility of distant relatives or close friends who could act as guardians should this prove necessary.

b. If she continues to drive despite counselling, gentle persuasion and perhaps a warning of possible police involvement, then serious consideration must be given to informing the Driver and Vehicle Licensing Centre (DVLC) in Swansea. Should you do this then be prepared to defend your position against a breach of confidentiality. You would be advised to contact your medical insurance agency for legal advice.

c. If she persists in driving then presumably you could inform the police on the grounds she was driving illegally (if her licence has been revoked by the DVLC). Once again, the issue of confidentiality is important, since informing the police would also constitute a breach of confidentiality.

d. If it can be argued that she is unsafe when she is driving in her car — as it would be possible to do in this example — then clearly she is not only endangering herself, but others. Thus, an option would be to ask a psychiatrist for advice regarding further management, though any question of 'a section' under the Mental Health Act of 1983, would not be seriously considered in this case.

Case 4

A 20-year-old man who is HIV positive, but previously well, has increasing shortness of breath and a dry cough. He has been becoming increasingly lethargic and is losing weight. The doctor suspects *Pneumocystis carinii* pneumonia (PCP) and informs the patient of this. The patient is upset and says that he does not wish to be treated.

17.4.1 Should the doctor treat him?

The simple answer to this is not without his consent. Providing the clinician feels that he has fully explained to the patient the likely diagnosis, the significance of it, and that if untreated it would be likely to worsen and to become so serious as to make the patient likely to die, then it is for the patient, providing he is sane, to make the decision about whether he accepts treatment or not. When cases such as this have been encountered previously in our unit, it is often the fear of invasive investigations and intravenous injections which is worrying the patient most of all. This, coupled with the possible loss of confidentiality if the patient is admitted, may lead to a compromise being reached, where the patient could remain as an outpatient, looked after at home and receive oral therapy. In mild cases of PCP, this may be an acceptable form of management and meet the patient's as well as the physician's requirements.

17.4.2 His parents feel very strongly that he should be treated. Does this make any difference?

None at all. Obviously if the patient consented to hold a discussion between himself, his family and the clinician, then this may be used to affect a mediation against his wish not to be treated. The onus is on the physician to satisfy himself that the patient clearly understands the pros and cons of treatment and their condition. Once he is satisfied with this, and that the patient is not psychiatrically unwell, then it is the patient's choice of whether to receive therapy or not. At the very least, the physician should set a further appointment to discuss the implications of the patient's decision with the patient, and if possible the patient's family and carers. The patient should also be assured that other medications which may make them more comfortable and relieve their symptoms would be offered, even if they decided against active treatment.

17.4.3 Over the next few days he becomes much more ill, confused and rambling. However, he says that he has changed his mind and wants to be treated. What should be done now?

In this particular case, it is likely that treatment would then be instigated. However, if the patient has set out his wishes and has left clear instructions, possibly in the form of a living will, that he is not to be treated and has given the name of a lover or next-of-kin to make decisions for him, then it is likely that the individual clinician would honour the patient's decisions. It goes without saying that every case should be treated on its merits, but such issues and especially the issues of living wills, may indeed help doctors to manage such contentious cases in future.

Case 5

A woman of 25 is found to be HIV positive. She admits to having many sexual partners and to using intravenous drugs recreationally.

17.5.1 Should her sexual partners be traced to warn them of the possibility of HIV infection?

Firstly, there is the question of whether any of her previous sexual partners or those she has had contact with sharing needles during injecting drug use, etc. can actually be contacted. If not, either because the patient does not know their names or current whereabouts, or does not wish to tell the clinician their identity, then no further action can be taken. Secondly, if it is possible to trace any of the contacts, it would be ideal that the patient herself, with her full knowledge and understanding of the issues concerned, was to make contact and suggest that they had a full health check-up. She should receive counselling around this event, as it may be both traumatic for her and risk her confidentiality of her own condition being breached. Many patients wish to take this risk for the benefit of those with whom they have had friendships and love affairs.

There is no evidence that the enforced coercion to obtain details of sexual partners, with consequent compulsory third party notification to those named about their risk of contracting HIV infection, has any beneficial effect whatsoever on the HIV transmission rate in a community. However, the benefits of voluntary schemes have been shown to be useful, especially in terms of identifying those who have been at risk of contracting HIV infection, and giving them sexual health education to try to reduce their lifestyle risks in future.

17.5.2 If her sexual partners are traced, what should they be told?

If the patient or a third party asks the contact to get in touch with an experienced health worker, then a full risk history for both HIV and other sexually acquired infections should be taken. The contact can be told that they have been in contact with somebody with an infection, but the name of the contact should not be given. It may be that this will be obvious to the patient concerned, and such an ethical issue should have been previously discussed with the individual original index patient. The contact should be offered a full range of tests, including an HIV test, with particular support and counselling being offered and post-test counselling also being available.

17.5.3 The woman refuses to inform the doctor as to whom her partners are. What should be done?

No action should be taken as it is unlikely that any contact tracing technique would work against the patient's wishes.

17.5.4 You suspect that she is using sex to pay for her drug habit. She is likely to continue to do this in the future and not engage in any safer sexual practices. What should be done?

The doctor may wish to confront the patient with his suspicions and to discuss her reasons for this. It may be that there are financial issues which might be relieved by help from the social services or voluntary charities. If there are other reasons besides the financial one, then this should be discussed with her and either counsellors and/or psychiatrists involved in the management of the case. In an extreme case, where the patient refused to give up unprotected sex, in Australia a prostitute was confined for the protection of others. As yet, no case such as this has occurred in the UK. If the prostitute insists that she always ensures that her clients use condoms, then the case becomes extremely difficult ethically. Although she knows she is HIV infected, she is insisting that she is giving all the possible protection to her clients that she would to a new sexual partner. The clients of this woman are placing themselves at risk despite having access to information about safer sex and issues surrounding HIV transmission, and therefore are equally as culpable.

Case 6

A man who admits to having sex with other men is found to be HIV antibody positive at your general practice. He is well. He informs the doctor that he is married. He says that he does not want his wife to know that he is positive. His wife is not registered with you.

17.6.1 Should his wife be informed?

This depends partly on whether he intends to continue having sex with his wife, whether she has ever been HIV antibody tested in the past and on the individual case. Clearly, if he says he hasn't had sex with his wife for 2 years, she had a negative HIV test 6 months ago, and he does not intend to have sex with her again, then there are less reasons to become involved. If this is not the case, then the clinician needs to give very great concern to this issue.

17.6.2 The patient says that he cannot suddenly start using condoms when having sex with his wife because she will suspect something. He will therefore have unprotected sex. Should his wife now be told?

If this is the case, then the doctor may wish to tell the patient that he feels this is an unsatisfactory state of affairs and that if the patient still wishes to be under his care, he will intervene by asking for an interview with both the wife and the husband, where he will precipitate discussion of the husband's condition. If the patient wishes to change doctors, that is then his right. Under such circumstances, it is likely that the patient may see his way to reducing his fears of the consequences for the sake of his wife.

17.6.3 The patient's wife registers at your general practice. She does not know that she is at risk. She appears to be anaemic and you take some blood. Would you do an HIV antibody test?

There would be absolutely no place for doing an HIV antibody test without the consent of the woman. This is because if a test was taken without her consent, there is no resolution of the initial dilemma as to whether to break her husband's confidence and reveal his HIV status. If the test result is negative, it is possible that either she is infected with the virus and is in the negative window phase of infection, or she remains uninfected but is still at continued risk of infection. If the result is positive, it is obviously too late to do anything about preventing her from acquiring HIV infection. It can therefore be seen that the dilemma is not resolved and the doctor is placed in the difficult position of possibly receiving a positive HIV test result on someone who is unaware that they have been tested.

However, it may be a good time to discuss with her the possibility of doing other blood tests, and in that context bring up the possibility of HIV testing. This may act as a handle for broaching any possible concerns that she may have about her husband's sexual activities or possible ill health.

17.6.4 To whom do you owe a duty of care?

Obviously, if both husband and wife are registered with your practice, the duty of care belongs to each of them as individuals. This obviously does not resolve the dilemma as to whether it is reasonable to inform the woman of her husband's HIV status without his consent. This dilemma has to be resolved by each individual practitioner, although many would feel that they were unable to withhold the information from the woman if her husband continued to keep her in the dark. It is possible that the dilemma may be resolved if he is told that you will inform his wife of his

HIV status, if he continues to refuse to, because of the duty of care that you owe her. This may provide the final piece of pressure required to encourage him to act responsibly.

There is no precedent as to how the courts would view the breach of confidentiality involved in such a case if the woman was informed without her husband's consent. The major defence unions in the UK have said that they would be happy to support a medical practitioner if they took this course of action and were subsequently prosecuted.

At the time of writing, there is a case unfolding in the USA where a medical practitioner is being sued, by someone who acquired HIV infection, for failing to inform that individual of their partner's HIV status.

Case 7

Peter, a 27-year-old gay man who has had AIDS for 3 years, wakes up one morning noticing that his eyesight is not normal. He phones his GP and asks for an appointment. The receptionist tells him that they are booked up until tomorrow.

17.7.1 Should the receptionist do anything else?

The implications of this question are obviously that any abnormality of vision in a patient such as Peter is a very serious complaint, and it would be hoped that he would be seen that day. Whether this would happen or not in reality depends to a certain extent on the structure of an individual general practice. Some practices would want such a complaint to be put through to either the doctor or the practice nurse for them to decide if they need to be seen that day. In some practices, the receptionist would be provided with a list of people who are potentially severely unwell to ensure that an appointment would be made for them.

It would be hoped that on most occasions Peter would be seen that day, as, if he does have cytomegalovirus (CMV) retinitis, 24 hours' delay could lead to marked and permanent deterioration in his vision. However, it has to be accepted that in an imperfect world, occasionally such a patient would slip through the net, especially if they lacked assertion during the phone call.

17.7.2 Peter goes to casualty and is discharged from the hospital 3 weeks later. He has CMV retinitis and requires intravenous treatment to stop his blindness. This involves giving a drug through a central line for 20 minutes, 5 times a week for the rest of his life. The hospital asks the GP to give some of the treatments. The GP refuses. Can he do this and do reasons have to be given?

If the letter of the GP's contract is followed, he may refuse to give any treatment or refuse to treat any patient once they are removed from his list without giving reason.

Assuming the GP does not wish to do this, there are two problems raised. Firstly, the fact that the doctor will have to take medical responsibility for giving a drug that he may be unfamiliar with and, secondly, the time involved in what is probably already a busy schedule.

In response to the first point, it would be hoped that the hospital would provide information about the administration, possible side-effects and necessary monitoring of ganciclovir or Foscarnet, depending on which one is prescribed. It would obviously be wrong to expect a GP to give a drug that they are not happy to administer.

In response to the second point, most patients who are on maintenance intravenous therapy for CMV will either administer the drug themselves or have it administered by a member of their family, their partner or one of their friends. As the GP is being asked to administer it, it is likely that Peter's vision has deteriorated to a degree where he is unable to self-administer, and that no alternative arrangements can be made on some occasions. As the prognosis of severe CMV retinitis is very poor, it is likely that the treatments will not go on for too long a period. It is possible that the only way Peter can be kept at home towards the end of his life is if some of the treatments are delivered by community health carers. With this in mind, we would always encourage GPs to look upon it as a very valuable use of their time. There are also many ways in which the inconvenience can be minimized, such as getting the patient to come down to the surgery, where the GP can see other patients in between setting up the infusion and taking it down, or supervising either the practice nurse or one of the local district nurses in giving the infusion.

17.7.3 Peter finds a new GP who is willing to help, but he asks the practice nurse to do it. She refuses for three reasons:
a. She does not have an intravenous certificate.
b. She does not like homosexuals.
c. She does not want to look after someone with AIDS.
Are any of these motives reasonable and could the district nurse use any of them?

To deal with part (a) first, a practice nurse is considered to be an employee of the GP, and he is therefore responsible for covering her for any procedures she undertakes during the course of her work. Therefore, an intravenous certificate is unnecessary. On a practical level, it would seem very unreasonable for a GP to insist that their practice nurse should give a treatment that they do not feel adequately educated to give. However, if the GP provides suitable training and support, there is no reason why the practice nurse should not give the treatments.

To deal with parts (b) and (c) together, the governing body of British nurses, the UKCC, have made it very clear in their internal ruling that all nurses are obliged by their professional regulations to provide whatever care is necessary for people with AIDS. It would also be unacceptable in their eyes for a nurse to refuse to treat anyone on the grounds of their race, religion or sexuality. It would seem sensible that if these excuses were given by the nurse for refusing to treat the patient, the employing GP should take the opportunity to educate his practice nurse about the possible modes of transmission of HIV. Her refusal to give the treatment because she does not like homosexuals would be viewed much more seriously in most people's eyes, and many practitioners would feel that this level of prejudice would cast doubt upon her suitability for continued employment.

In the case of the district nurse, the answers are exactly the same, except for the fact that a district nurse is the employee of the local health authority, and therefore will almost inevitably need a certificate of intravenous training before she can administer drugs in this way.

17.7.4 When Peter comes to the surgery the receptionist thinks he looks rather tired. She asks a patient to give up her chair in the waiting room for him, saying 'you don't mind, do you? He has got AIDS you know'. What needs to be done now?

Obviously the first thing that needs to be done in such a situation is to address the immediate effects of this statement on Peter. To this end, it would seem reasonable to take him into the consulting room and apologize unreservedly for the breach in confidentiality, while obviously pointing out that it is probable that the receptionist was actually trying to help him. Any further action as far as Peter is concerned depends on his response.

What action to take with the receptionist will largely depend on her quality of work up until that moment. Most receptionists' contracts will have a confidentiality clause written into them and breach of this will be seen as grounds for instant dismissal. Whether this course of action is taken or not, is likely to depend on whether the receptionist is an efficient, invaluable member of the practice staff, or someone whom the practice have been looking for an excuse to get rid of for some time.

18. Practical information and further reading

The first part of this chapter aims to provide some information about both voluntary and statutory services which may be helpful when managing patients with HIV infection and AIDS. The list of services given is far from exhaustive. It also has a marked bias towards London-based services. This is partly in reflection of the concentration of people affected by HIV infection and AIDS in this area, and partly because many nationwide organizations have their headquarters in London. A more extensive picture of available services, particularly for areas outside London, can be gained by consulting the National AIDS Manual or referring to your local HIV Coordinator.

The National AIDS Manual is a three-volume tome which is regularly updated. It provides full information on all facilities available for people with HIV infection, including statutory and voluntary services, treatment centres and research trials available throughout the country. It is likely that the health advisor at your local Genitourinary Medicine Clinic will have access to it. Every District Health Authority has a designated AIDS Coordinator who should be able to provide information about local services.

USEFUL SERVICES AND ADDRESSES

ACET (AIDS Care Education and Training)
PO Box 1323
London W5 5TF
Tel: (081) 840 7879
ACET is a church-based charity which aims to give practical help to people with AIDS. The help provided includes home care and grants to help pay household bills, buy equipment and pay for holidays. The home care services are currently largely restricted to the London area, but the charity is looking to expand to include other areas in the near future, Edinburgh and Brighton being considered high priorities.

Bethany
St Mary's Road
Bodmin
Cornwall PL31 1NF
Tel: (0208) 79035
Bethany offers rest and respite care for people with HIV and AIDS.

BHAN (Black HIV/AIDS Network)
111 Devonport Road
London W12 8PB
Tel: (081) 742 9223 (Helpline)
      (081) 749 2828 (Administration)
Services provided by BHAN include support for black people with HIV
infection and also black people who work in the field. They are developing
specific groups such as the South-East Asian HIV/AIDS support group.

Blackliners
PO Box 74
London SW12 9JY
Tel: (081) 673 1695
      (071) 738 5274 (Helpline)
This organization has been set up to target HIV/AIDS information
towards black and Asian communities. The services they provide include
helpline leaflets, posters, counselling and support groups.

Body Positive
51B Philbeach Gardens
Earls Court
London SW5 9EB
Tel: (071) 373 9124 (Helpline)
      (071) 835 1045 (Centre)
      (071) 490 1225 (Women's line)
      (071) 370 1066 (Small grants)
Body Positive was the original group set up for people who are HIV
antibody positive by people who are HIV antibody positive. There are
now many different regional offices in different cities and towns
throughout the country, and it is also an international organization with
branches in many different countries. The headquarters in London offer
a wide variety of services which include a drop-in centre, advice sessions
on such topics as welfare rights, health and legal matters, counselling and
therapy groups, support evenings and it produces a newsletter. The
London office will also be able to provide information on regional Body
Positive groups.

CARA (Care and Resources of people affected by AIDS/HIV)
The Basement
178 Lancaster Road
London W11 2UU
Tel: (071) 792 8299
This group aims to enable the church to share in a creative response to AIDS. It offers spiritual, emotional and practical support to people affected in any way by the virus.

Catholic AIDS Link
PO Box 646
London E9 6QP
Tel: (081) 986 0807
Catholic AIDS Link offers spiritual, emotional and practical support to those affected by HIV and AIDS, and training, counselling and networking facilities for staff.

City Roads (Crisis Intervention) Ltd
358 City Road
London EC1V 2PY
Tel: (071) 278 8671/8672 (Crisis line)
     (071) 837 2772/2773 (Administration)
City Roads is a short-term centre for chaotic drug users offering detox, medical and social work support. It operates a nationwide catchment.

Crusaid
21A Upper Tachbrook Street
London SW1V 1SN
Tel: (071) 834 7566
Crusaid is an AIDS fundraising charity which, as well as providing larger grants for community and public needs such as outpatient clinics, will also help individuals in financial need.

FACTS (Foundation for AIDS Counselling Treatment and Support)
Between 23/25 Western Park
Crouch End
London N8 9SY
Tel: (081) 348 9195
Services provided for people with HIV infection include a medical outpatients clinic, advice sessions, counselling and complementary therapies. There is also a gym available for use by clients.

The Food Chain
c/o BM Food Chain
London WC1N 3XX
Tel: (081) 801 4286
The Food Chain delivers a weekly Sunday three-course meal to people
with AIDS in the Greater London area. The meals are specially tailored
to meet the needs of people with AIDS.

Gay Bereavement Project
c/o Unitarian Rooms
Hoop Lane
London NW11 8BS
Tel: (081) 455 8894
This is a gay organization offering bereavement counselling, support and
help with practical problems following bereavement. It can also give
advice on funeral arrangements.

The Griffin Project
6 Penywern Road
Earls Court
London SW5
Tel: (071) 373 9826
The Griffin Project is a residential nursing home for people with HIV
infection and a history of drug use. Services provided include respite
care, convalescent care, post acute care, drug management and palliative
care.

Immunity
260A Kilburn Lane
London W10 4BA
Tel: (081) 968 8909
As well as offering legal advice and welfare rights advice to people with
HIV infection, Immunity also conducts research into social, medical and
legal aspects of HIV infection, and produces educational material and
information leaflets.

Landmark
47A Tulse Hill
London SW2 2TN
Tel: (081) 678 6686
Services offered by the Landmark include nursing, consultation, massage,
acupuncture, transportation service and social work support, as well as a
drop-in centre for people living with HIV and AIDS.

LEAN (London East AIDS Network)
35 Romford Road
Stratford
London E15 4LY
Tel: (081) 519 9545
This is a voluntary group which provides support services for people with HIV in East London. It can also offer small grants and produces leaflets on HIV and AIDS in a variety of Asian languages.

The London Lighthouse
111–117 Lancaster Road
London W11 1QT
Tel: (071) 792 1200
The London Lighthouse provides a wide range of different services which include the residential unit which offers convalescent, respite and terminal care, and a day centre where nursing care can be offered to people with HIV and AIDS. They have an informal drop-in area with a cafe, information services, social activities, counselling, support groups and complementary therapies. They also offer an outreach home support facility.

Mainlines
PO Box 125
London SW9 8EF
Tel: (071) 274 4000 ext 354
Services are provided for drug users and ex-drug users who are HIV antibody positive or who are worried about issues concerning HIV infection. Services include a helpline, counselling, advice and information.

Mildmay Mission Hospital
Hackney Road
London E2 7NA
Tel: (071) 739 2331
This is an independent, Christian charitable hospital in the East End of London, providing care for people with AIDS and for young disabled people. It has a specialist AIDS hospice unit and continuing care unit which provide respite, rehabilitive, convalescent and terminal care. Counselling support, day care and home care back-up are also available.

Milestone House
113 Oxgangs Road North
Edinburgh EH14 1EB
Tel: (031) 441 6989
This continuing care unit is specifically for people living in the Lothian area. Respite, convalescent and palliative care are offered.

National AIDS Helpline
Tel: (0800) 567 123
This a free 24-hour national helpline which offers advice and information
on any aspect of HIV infection to anyone calling.

The Open Door
Tel: (0273) 605706
Open Door is in Brighton. As well as providing a drop-in service and a
daily meal for people with HIV and AIDS, people may also come for a
week's holiday or convalescence.

The Patrick House
17 Rivercourt Road
London W6
Tel: (081) 846 9117
Patrick House is a residential nursing home for people with brain impairment related to HIV and AIDS. It is the first such institution of its kind
in Europe.

Positive Partners
Suite 305
Panther House
38 Mount Pleasant
London WC1X 0AP
Tel: (071) 278 2232
This is self-help group for all people directly affected by HIV, including
people with HIV and AIDS, their partners, friends, carers and families.
Services include support groups, counselling, complementary and alterna-
tive therapies, advice on housing, financial, drug, medical and legal
problems, and small grants for those who are HIV antibody positive and
in need.

Positive Youth
c/o Body Positive
51 Philbeach Gardens
Earls Court
London SW5 9EB
Tel: (071) 373 7547
Positive Youth is a group for young men and women under the age of 25
years living with HIV and AIDS.

Positively Children
Suite 305
Panther House
38 Mount Pleasant
London WC1X 0AP
Tel: (071) 278 2232
This is a group set up under the auspices of Positive Partners for people
under the age of 18 with HIV infection, or who have a parent or guardian
with HIV infection, and also for parents of children with HIV and AIDS.

Positively Women
5 Sebastian Street
London EC1V 0HE
Tel: (071) 490 5515
A wide range of free and strictly confidential counselling and support
services are provided to women with AIDS and HIV. These include
support groups, telephone and/or face to face counselling and a buddying
service.

The Red Admiral Project
51A Philbeach Gardens
Earls Court
London SW5 9EB
Tel: (071) 835 1495
Intensive counselling and/or support can be provided for people affected
by HIV infection, their partners, lovers, family and friends.

The Riverhouse
Furnival Gardens
by Rutland Grove
Hammersmith
London W6
Tel: (081) 563 0343
The Riverhouse is a drop-in centre for people with HIV and AIDS.

Streetwise
Flat 3B Langham Mansions
London SW5 9UP
Tel: (071) 370 0406
     (071) 378 8860 (Helpline)
Streetwise provides help for young, male sex workers. Services include
refuge, day care, education and support.

The Sussex AIDS Centre
PO Box 17
Brighton BN2 5NQ
Tel: (0273) 571 660 (Helpline)
    (0273) 608 511
Services provided by the Centre include a home care team, a fund for medical equipment which is not available on the NHS, counselling, social work and occupational therapy.

The Sussex Beacon
Bevendean Road
Brighton BN2 4DE
Tel: (0273) 694 222
The Sussex Beacon opened as a continuing care unit for people with HIV and AIDS in Brighton at the end of 1992. It offers respite care, convalescent care and palliative care.

The Terrence Higgins Trust
52/54 Grays Inn Road
London WC1X 8LT
Tel: (071) 831 0330
    (071) 242 1010 (Helpline)
The Terrence Higgins Trust is the largest AIDS/HIV charity in Britain. Services which it provides include a helpline, buddying, counselling, legal helpline, welfare advice, hardship grants, prison visits and support groups.

Threshold Housing Advice Centre   126 Uxbridge Road
91–99 Tooting High Street   London W12
London SW17   Tel: (081) 749 2925
Tel: (081) 682 0322
This group will provide help for anyone with HIV infection who is facing any sort of housing problem.

GUIDE TO FURTHER READING

Adler M W (ed) 1988 Diseases in the homosexual male. Bloomsbury Series in Clinical Science, Springer Verlag, London
Adler M W (ed) 1990 ABC of AIDS (2E). British Medical Association, London
Ansary M A, Hira S K, Bayley A C et al 1989 AIDS in the tropics. Wolfe Publications, London
Cohen P T, Sande M A, Volberding P A (eds) 1990 The AIDS knowledge base. M A Medical Society, USA
Hopp J W, Rogers E A (eds) 1989 AIDS and the allied health professions. Davis Co, Philadelphia
Johnstone F D (ed) 1992 Clinical obstetrics and gynaecology. Bailliere Tindall, London
Joshi V V (ed) 1990 Pathology of AIDS and other manifestations of HIV infection. Igaku-Shoin, New York

Kotler D P (ed) 1992 Gastrointestinal and nutritional manifestations of the acquired immunodeficiency syndrome. Raven Press, New York

Kramer L 1989 Reports from the holocaust, the making of an AIDS activist. St Martins Press, New York

Miller D 1987 Living with AIDS and HIV. MacMillan Education Ltd, UK

Reamer F G (ed) 1991 AIDS and ethics. Columbia University Press, New York

Sande M A, Volberding P A (eds) 1990 The medical management of AIDS (2E). W B Saunders Company, Philadelphia

Sande M A (ed) 1992 HIV infection and AIDS. Current Science, London

Strang J, Stimson G (eds) 1990 AIDS and drug misuse. Routledge, London

Youle M, Clarbour J, Wade P et al 1988 AIDS: therapeutics in HIV disease. Churchill Livingstone, London

JOURNALS TO BE CONSULTED

AIDS
AIDS Care
Annals of Internal Medicine
British Medical Journal
Current Opinion in Infectious Diseases
Genitourinary Medicine
International Journal of STD and AIDS
Journal of AIDS
Journal of Immunology
Journal of Virology
Lancet
New England Journal of Medicine

Index